KineBody™

Functional Strength Development for men and women

Edgardo Aponte

Disclaimer:
The exercises described in this book may be too strenuous for some people. Please consult your physician before beginning this or any other physical training regimen.

Nothing within this book intends to constitute an explanation of the use of any product or the carrying out of any procedure or process introduced by or within any material. Information contained in this book is not a substitute for professional medical advice, health care services or a medical exam. Nothing in this book is to be interpreted as a general or specific recommendation for a specific treatment plan, product, exercise regimen or course of action. Consult your doctor before using any exercise device or program. Do not perform any activity if you have any special medical condition. Only your doctor or a qualified medical professional can provide you with advice or recommendations for an individual ailment, treatment or problem.

Use this book at your own risk. Failure to follow instructions and/or using the information in this book in any way other than its intended use could result in injury. The reader understands the risk associated with using the information contained in this book, and the purchaser understands the risk associated with following instructions from this book.

The author and publisher of this book are not responsible in any manner whatsoever for any injury which may occur through reading and following the instructions herein.

The information contained in this book is for educational and informational purposes only. The author and publisher make no guarantees or claims as to the effectiveness or accuracy of anything presented in this book. By purchasing and/or reading this book you agree that the author, publisher or any party involved in creating, producing or delivering this book shall not be liable for any damages, including without limitation, direct, incidental, consequential, indirect or punitive damages, arising out of access to, use of or inability to use the information presented in this book, or any errors or omissions in the content thereof.

KineBody: Functional Strength Development for Men and Women

ISBN 1-4196-7596-6

Contents

Contents

Acknowledgment

To my wonderful wife, Rosanna. For her patience, support, and assistance in the creation
of this manuscript, I thank her and appreciate her each and every day.
To my parents. For their support of all my endeavors.

Introduction

I became involved with physical fitness way back in 1986. This was the year I left my home of New York City to study at Penn State. Penn State seemed like a world away from the busy and crowded streets of New York City, and it was also home to one of the biggest college martial arts clubs in the country at the time.

I joined the Isshinryu Karate Club shortly after I arrived at Penn State and fell in love with the martial arts instantly. Though I suffered through several weeks of soreness, I persevered and found myself practicing five to seven days per week, sometimes for three or more hours at a time. My workout sessions varied. Sometimes I would work on kata – prearranged fighting forms - designed to teach certain aspects of self-defense and to help train the body in attributes such as speed, coordination and balance. Other times I would spar with other classmates, drill individual techniques over and over again for hours at a time, or hit the punching bags.

Throughout my years at Penn State, I steadily progressed and earned my 2nd degree black belt, I trained hundreds of students in the art of Isshinryu karate, and even placed 2nd at the 1988 Isshinryu World Karate Championships. But it didn't stop there. Though I majored in liberal arts, my fascination with the martial arts peaked my interest in other aspects of physical fitness. Therefore, I took several courses in exercise science and athletic training, and also worked towards earning CPR certification. The result of years of martial arts training and coursework in exercise science and athletic training was the ability to do 70 push ups within 60 seconds, run 2 miles in under 14 minutes, maintain the flexibility to do a complete split, have body fat of 6%, and become one of the most technically proficient black belts of the Isshinryu Karate Club during the late 1980's and early 1990's.

In 1991 I left the comfort of my life at Penn State. I traveled half way around the world to make my new home in Taipei, Taiwan. While there, I would teach English, travel throughout Asia, train with some of the most gifted martial artists of their day, and learn some of the more exotic martial arts of the time.

Though I lived in Taiwan for only one year, I had the pleasure of visiting such wonderful places such as South Korea, Okinawa, mainland China, Hong Kong and Macao. During this time, I also took the opportunity for intense training with karate masters in

Okinawa, kung fu practitioners in China, a shaolin fighting instructor in Taiwan, and a relocated Muay Thai boxer from Thailand. My training was intense, sometimes brutal, but well worth the experience of a lifetime

Once I returned to the States, I pursued a more traditional life, became a computer technician, but never lost my fascination with the martial arts or interest in physical fitness. Throughout the 1990's and early 2000's, I studied various other forms of martial arts such as kali, arnis, jiu-jitsu, sambo, Russian martial art, and Jeet Kune Do. At the same time, I continued to practice Isshinryu, pursued further training in Muay Thai, and wrote countless articles for some of the more popular martial arts publications at the time.

Sometime in 2005, I came to the realization that throughout my years of involvement in martial arts and physical fitness, one variable stayed constant – the ability to train anywhere, anytime, and without the need for any equipment. This lead to a new passion to design a system of physical fitness, physical culture, and wellness that would allow anyone the ability to train at any time, in virtually any place. The freedom I experienced while traveling, yet still being able to train and stay physically fit without the need for expensive equipment or even a roof over my head was something I wanted to capture under the umbrella of one system. Through decades of training and years of experience, I have devised a system for the average person. Something everyone can grab a hold of, take it with them anywhere, and call it their own. This system and approach has come to be called **KineBody™**.

*T*hough I have many years of martial arts and physical fitness experience under my belt, I still consider myself just an average guy. My interests include computers, electronic gadgets, traveling, martial arts, and physical fitness. I read about these topics through books, magazines, and the Internet. From time-to-time I also like to take courses, classes, or training sessions in some of these topics. This is why, in 2006, I decided to take an in-depth curriculum in becoming a personal trainer through the excellent Equinox Fitness Clubs. Though I hold fitness clubs and other gyms in very high regard (after all, they are doing what they can to perpetuate good fitness habits), I still couldn't shake the idea that all gyms need to generate revenue by convincing current and prospective clients that a gym membership, free weights, resistance machines, treadmills, cycles, stair masters, and even stretching racks are necessary items for maintaining overall health and well-being. Though it's nice to have choices, and for more sport specific training, such as bodybuilding or Olympic style lifting, equipment is absolutely necessary, for the vast majority of the average population, staying in shape does not require the need for expensive equipment, time away from home, or the perpetual expenditure of monthly gym memberships. In a many, overwhelmingly large, number of cases, all that's needed is your own body, a small amount of floor space, a couple of pieces of furniture and an investment in time...that's it.

I wanted to devise a system of physical fitness and wellness for the average person. Whether you are turned-off by going to a gym, hate working out in large groups, or are intimidated at the idea of training in a public setting, you need to know that you have options. One of these options (amongst many), is my system, which I call **KineBody**.

Pronounced (**kin-ay-body**), **KineBody** comes from the word *kinesiology*, which means "the study of human movement," with *kine* referring to motion. Therefore, **KineBody** is another way of saying body movement, body motion, or body in motion. It's that simple; your body in motion, devoid of all those mental distractions that can come from other people, loud music blasting in a gym, complicated equipment, or simply standing around waiting to use a favorite piece of equipment in a crowded gym.

The catch phrase I like to use is **KineBody: your body ... your gym™**. It really is just that simple. And just like other forms of exercise such as yoga, pilates, or martial arts, **KineBody** is a system of **functional body development** with structure and organization.

By **functional body development**, I mean training your body, or regions of your body, as a unit. Most of the exercises, postures, drills, and skills performed through **KineBody** are designed to avoid muscle isolation. Though a very small percentage of the exercises are considered isolation exercises, I have tried to minimize the use of these exercises and concentrated on utilizing the body as one functional unit to achieve a desired result. In much the same way that climbing a set of stairs or lifting a heavy box off the ground requires the use of many muscle groups, joints, and tendons working together, so does the **functional body development** approach of **KineBody**. Training in this approach is much more realistic in terms of real-world function, than trying to isolate your biceps by performing a biceps curl or trying to isolate your quads by performing a leg extension. These isolation exercises have their place (and do develop strength in those isolated areas), but they do nothing towards teaching the body to react in real-world situations.

As a system of **functional body development**, **KineBody** is divided into four training categories that work together to achieve tremendous fitness benefits for the average person. By the average person, I mean that you, me, or anyone else can achieve results by incorporating **KineBody** into your fitness routine. Don't be fooled though. As this book will show, even those in tremendous physical shape will find something challenging and worth their valuable time and effort.

With this in mind, the four training categories are as follows:

- **Functional Strength Development**: the use of bodyweight exercises, leverage, and maximum tension to develop strength, conditioning, and endurance
- **Functional Flexibility & Joint Mobility**: muscular stretching and joint mobility drills to develop injury free movement throughout a greater range of motion
- **Functional Balance & Coordination**: incorporating static postures, footwork, and animated body mechanics to enhance balance and body awareness
- **Functional Sport Specificity**: putting it all together to enhance sport specific skills. In my case, I like to call this category **Functionally Applied Martial Arts** because I use the above categories to enhance attributes related to benefiting my martial arts skills

Functional Strength Development

*B*y the title of this book, you have no doubt figured out what category of **KineBody's** training system we are concentrating on. The focus of this book will be on **Functional Strength Development (FSD)**. By using **KineBody's FSD** approach, we will use our own bodyweight to achieve impressive results in building lean muscle mass that will give us more strength and or endurance in a wide variety of activities related to everyday function or applied to the sport of your choosing.

KineBody's FSD provides a whole range of benefits because using your own bodyweight in ways that stress the muscles and increase tension during a particular range of motion provides the necessary stimulus for muscle fiber growth. Now, I'm not saying that someone using **KineBody's FSD** approach is going to become a world-class bodybuilder, but what I am saying is that any weight-bearing exercise that produces the correct stimulus can encourage and will facilitate muscle growth. As we will see shortly, weight-bearing exercises in the correct set/rep scheme can produce results in power/strength, hypertrophy (muscle growth), or endurance. As well as building strong, lean muscle, any weight-bearing exercise promotes good bone density. And, because muscle burns more calories than fat, having more muscle on your bodyframe helps to burn more calories throughout the day, even during rest. Though conflicting reports state that one pound of muscle burns from as little as 6 calories per day, to as high as 50 calories per day, one pound of fat generally burns only about 2 calories per day.

Lastly, **KineBody's FSD** can make for a short, time-efficient training session that not only provides the muscle-strengthening, bone-density building, fat-burning workout we want, but also gives us the cardiovascular benefits of typical cardio workouts like jogging or bicycling. Why? The **complex** (also known as circuit training). The complex involves doing several different exercises, one after the other, with little rest in between. For example, do push ups, run-in-place during the rest period, do pull ups, run-in-place during the rest period, do squats, run-in-place during the rest period. Now repeat that one entire complex for three or four sets, and what you have is an intense, 20-minute session that satisfies your cardio and strength routine in one shot.

KineBody's FSD aims to facilitate the above results by making use of the *closed kinetic chain* and *compound* exercises. Let's take a quick look at what exactly the closed kinetic chain is.

Exercises can be classified into *open kinetic chain* or *closed kinetic chain* movements. Open kinetic chain exercises are designed to isolate a particular muscle by performing the exercise using only one joint. In open kinetic chain movements, the end of the chain of movement is open or free. Examples of open kinetic chain exercises are biceps curls where the flexion and extension of the elbow joint serve to contract the biceps muscles in such a way that only the biceps region of the arm is stressed when a load is applied throughout the range of motion. The same can be said about the leg extension, where the knee is flexed and extended so the quadriceps muscles are isolated as a load is applied throughout the range of motion. Though open kinetic chain exercises have value and serve a purpose, they use single-joint movements that provide very little advantage when it comes to functional body development.

Functional body development, on the other hand, is training that requires the integration of balance, coordination, and muscular stability during the application of muscular force. This type of training relies heavily on the use of closed kinetic chain, multi-joint movements that require compound exercises using multiple muscle groups. Unlike open kinetic chain movements, the closed kinetic chain's movement is fixed against an object that supports the body's weight such as the floor or chin up bar. Closed kinetic chain, functional training more closely resembles human movement, and provides for a more functional type of strength. This translates into better body performance during daily activities and reduces problems caused due to a lack of proper body awareness. Stair climbing is a perfect example of a closed kinetic chain, multi-joint, compound exercise. The stair is the object that closes the kinetic chain. By flexing and extending at both the hip and knee joint, we are utilizing a multi-joint movement that works as a compound exercise stressing multiple muscle groups including the muscles of the buttocks (glutes), front of the thighs (quadriceps), and also involves the hip flexors and back of the thighs (hamstrings).

Now that we have a good understanding of the benefits involved in *KineBody's FSD* approach to functional body development, we are almost ready to dive into the dozens of exercises presented in this book. I say almost, because we have just three more topics to discuss as prerequisites to beginning an exercise program using *KineBody's FSD* approach.

First, we need to address the principle of ***antagonistic muscle groups***, or opposite motion. Antagonistic muscles are muscles that perform the exact opposite motion in relation to each other. Usually, the muscle in the front of your body performs an opposite movement in relation to the muscle immediately behind it. This is just a generalization meant to simplify the explanation. Another way to think about antagonistic muscle groups is by example. For example, the biceps are a group of muscles in the front of your upper arm that allow you to bend (flex) the elbow so your hand can come up near your shoulder. The antagonistic movement is the extension (straightening the arm) caused by the antagonistic muscle located behind your upper arm, the triceps.

Anytime you train one muscle group, you should train the antagonistic muscle group, generally within the same week. Train your abdominals/lower back in the same week; train your chest/upper back in the same week; train your biceps/triceps in the same week; etc... This approach produces balanced muscle development throughout the body and can reduce injuries, or posture issues that come with over-training one antagonistic muscle group and neglecting the opposite antagonistic muscle group.

In terms of ***KineBody's FSD*** approach and the use of the closed kinetic chain, multi-joint, compound exercise concepts, we are going to think about muscle development in terms of movement instead of individual muscle groups. Therefore, we will work antagonistic movement patterns. All we need to remember is that **pushing** is antagonistic to **pulling**. So, in whatever plane of motion we perform a pushing exercise, we must also perform a pulling exercise in the same plane of motion, in order to properly work antagonistic muscles. A good example of the push/pull principle is the hand stand push up vs the standard pull up or chin up. If, during your week of training, you perform hand stand push ups, then at some point during that week you need to perform the exact opposite motion and do pull ups/chin ups. If you perform standard push ups, you need to also perform some sort of horizontal based pull ups. The only exception to this rule is when performing some sort of leg-pressing, such as squats, because no real type of opposite leg pulling exercise that adequately performs a load bearing opposite movement is feasible.

Secondly, we will touch on the concept of ***periodization***. Simply put, periodization means changing your workout routine. The best workout routine in the world can be thrown out the window in about 4-6 weeks. Why? Because over this period of time, your body will adapt to the routine and no longer make maximum gains from the routine. Even if you no longer wish to get bigger, stronger, faster, or leaner, periodization prevents boredom, may prevent overuse injuries, it gives your body a recovery period from the same exercise, and gives you a fresh outlook and maintains mental interest by trying something new and different. But, if you wish to continue making improvements in your physical attributes, periodization is an absolute must.

You can change your routine by simply changing the types of exercises you do, the order in which you do the exercises, the days of the week in which you train, the rest period between exercises, the amount of repetitions per exercise, or the amount of weight used for each exercise. In terms of the bodyweight exercises used in *Kinebody*, we can change the amount of weight (or load) placed on an exercise by, say, working from the standard two-arm push up to the one-arm push up, or by elevating the feet to place more of your weight over your upper back. With over **60 types** of exercises and variations presented in this book alone, you will be at no shortage for creating a variety of challenging routines. *KineBody's* unique approach to overloading a particular exercise comes from adjusting the amount of bodyweight placed over or under the muscle groups of interest, changing the leverage in order to make the exercise more difficult, and a combination of the two to create maximum tension on the targeted muscle groups. All this serves to provide for near endless possibilities in the types of challenging routines you can come up with.

Finally, we can discuss the different results based on the type of load (weight) placed on a particular training routine. Performing an exercise through a range of motion is considered a **repetition**. Performing that exercise for multiple repetitions until you come to almost complete muscular fatigue (the point where you can do maybe just one more repetition or perhaps none) is called a **set**. Performing various combinations of reps and sets can produce the following physical attributes:

- **Muscular endurance**: being able to perform a relatively high number of repetitions with a lower weight
- **Hypertrophy**: increasing muscle mass and size by lifting a higher weight for a lower number of repetitions
- **Power/Maximum Strength**: developing the power to lift a very large weight for a very small amount of repetitions

Depending on the attributes you want to develop, you can use the following chart:

Weight	Attribute	Repetitions	# of Sets
Light	Endurance	12 - 20	1 - 3
Moderate	Hypertrophy	8 - 12	1 - 6
Heavy	Power/Strength	1 - 8	1 - 5

Now remember, lifting **any** type of weight, whether it is with dumbbells, barbells, using resistance machines, or *KineBody's* bodyweight exercises can produce any of the above attributes as long as a state of fatigue (or near fatigue) is reached during each set using the prescribed repetitions above. Rest periods in between sets can range from 30 seconds for endurance training, up to 2 minutes for hypertrophy training, to as high as 2 – 5 minutes for power training. Even though many people don't associate bodyweight strength training with hypertrophy, just remember that if you find an exercise where you can only perform 8 to 12 repetitions before reaching muscular fatigue, and you perform this exercise over 1 to 6 sets, say twice per week, you will, no doubt, gain muscle mass and achieve hypertrophy. Rest assured, *KineBody's FSD* approach contains many exercises in this book that will challenge many people trying to achieve physical attributes in the chart above.

Now we can finally get to work, experiment with the exercises in this book, and create varied training routines to help us in achieving the health results we want. Below are just a few tips to get you started; some things to keep in mind and consider as you work your way to better health with *KineBody*.

- ✔ If you have been out of shape for some time, see a doctor first and start slowly. 2 to 3 days per week with 30 minute sessions should be plenty for the first few weeks
- ✔ Workout 3 – 4 days per week for endurance; 2 – 3 days/week for hypertrophy; 2 days/week for power
- ✔ If it hurts, don't do it, or see a doctor
- ✔ Get lots of sleep and eat low fat, low sugar, nutrient rich foods
- ✔ Strength development sessions should not exceed 60 minutes (30 to 60 minutes is plenty)
- ✔ Lastly, get yourself a pedometer and walk 10,000 steps/day 5 – 7 days/week (this can be done throughout the day; it doesn't have to happen in one session)

Perfect Push Up Progression

Standard 4 – Point Push Ups

Starting Position

1. Begin with your hands flat on the floor about shoulder width apart at chest level
2. Feet are together (or up to 6 inches apart), toes and balls of the feet touching the floor
3. The starting position requires that your arms be extended, and body be perfectly straight from head-to-ankles

Execution

1. Lower yourself towards the floor keeping several tips in mind:
   a. keep your elbows near your ribs (either touching your sides or up to just a few inches away) as this is a more functional way of applying a pushing motion
   b. keep your body in a straight line from head-to-ankles
   c. inhale as you lower yourself
2. Stop when your chin is within one inch from the floor
3. As you push away from the floor, extend your arms, exhale, return to the starting position
4. Repeat for a desired amount of repetitions per set

Body Parts Involved

This exercise will primarily work the muscle groups in the:
1. chest (pectoral muscles)
2. front of the shoulder (anterior deltoid muscle)
3. back of the upper arms (triceps)

Variations

1. **Wide-Grip 4 – Point Push Ups**
   a. hands are about 1 ½ to 2 shoulder widths apart at chest level
   b. elbows stay away from your sides as much as possible during execution
   c. wide-grip push ups place greater emphasis on the chest (pectoral muscles)
2. **Diamond 4 – Point Push Ups**
   a. hands are close together, at chest level, with tips of index fingers touching and tips of thumbs touching
   b. elbows stay close to your sides
   c. diamond push ups place greater emphasis on the back of the upper arms (triceps)

Note: To place more of your bodyweight over your arms, you may elevate both feet by placing them on steps of progressively increasing height, a chair, or couch. This effectively increases the weight you must push off the floor resulting in greater strength and muscle mass gains when utilized with the appropriate repetitions per set scheme.

Standard 4 – Point Push Ups

1

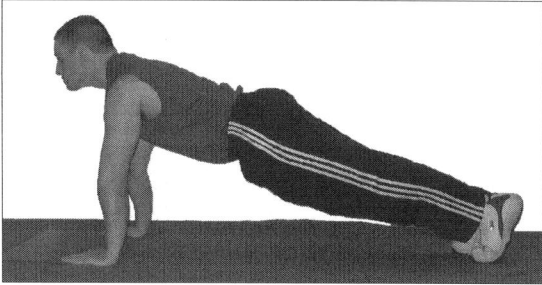

1a

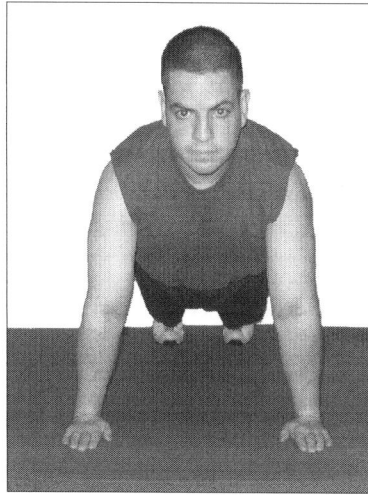

2

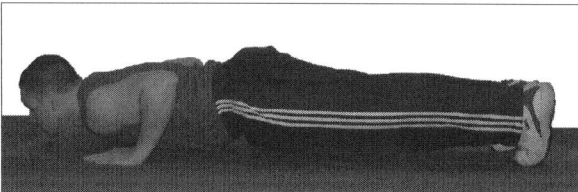

2a

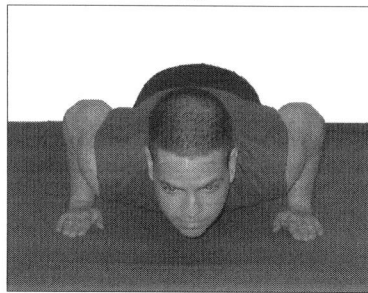

Wide Grip

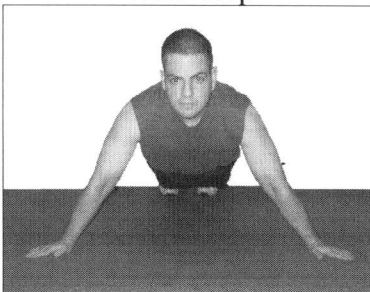

Diamond

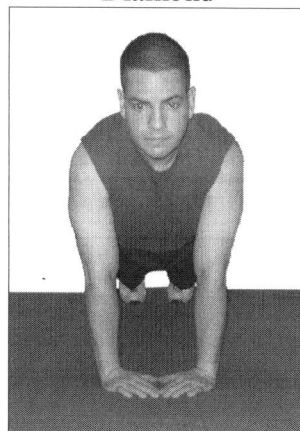

Side-to-Side, Top Starting, 4 – Point Push Ups

Starting Position

1. Begin with your hands flat on the floor about shoulder width apart at chest level
2. Feet are together (or up to 6 inches apart), toes and balls of the feet touching the floor
3. The starting position requires that your arms be extended, and body be perfectly straight from head-to-ankles

Execution

1. Shift your body weight (without moving your hands or feet) so it is over your right arm
2. Lower yourself towards the floor with most of your weight over your right arm
   a. keep your elbows near your ribs (either touching your sides or up to just a few inches away) as this is a more functional way of applying a pushing motion
   b. keep your body in a straight line from head-to-ankles
   c. inhale as you lower yourself
3. Stop when the right side of your chest touches your right hand
4. As you push away from the floor, use your right arm for the majority of the pushing, using your left only for assistance, extend your arms, exhale, return to the top starting position
5. Shift your body weight so it is over your left arm and repeat the motion over your left side (when you have done a repetition once on the right and once on the left, this is considered just ONE complete repetition)
6. Repeat for a desired amount of repetitions per set

Body Parts Involved

This exercise works the same muscle groups as the standard 4 – point push up (chest – pectoral muscles, front of shoulder – anterior deltoid muscle, back of the upper arms - triceps) except that greater demands are placed on the side you happen to be leaning on.

Note: To place more of your bodyweight over your arms, you may elevate both feet by placing them on steps of progressively increasing height, a chair, or couch. This effectively increases the weight you must push off the floor resulting in greater strength and muscle mass gains when utilized with the appropriate repetitions per set scheme.

Side-to-Side, Top Starting, 4 – Point Push Ups

1

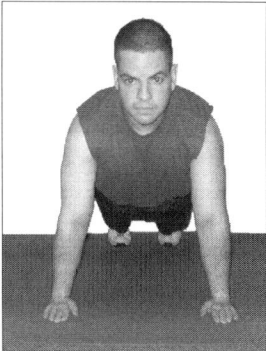

2

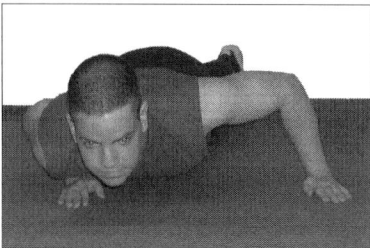

3

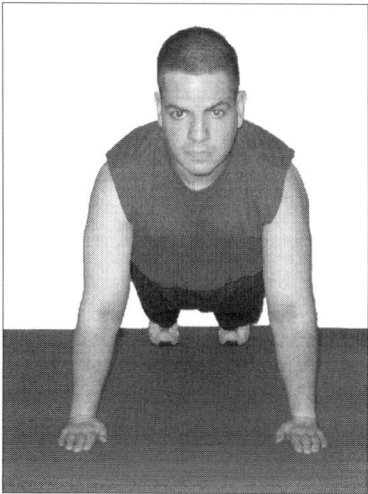

4

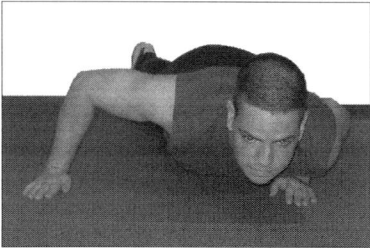

5

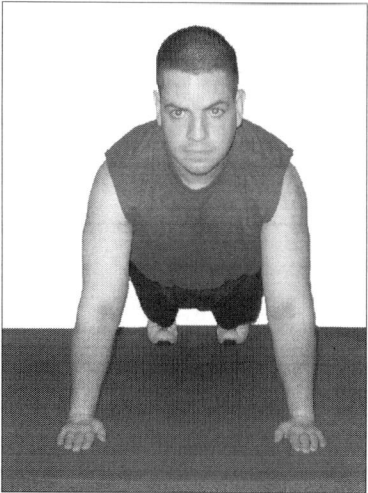

Side-to-Side, Bottom Starting, 4 – Point Push Ups

Starting Position

1. Begin with your hands flat on the floor about shoulder width apart at chest level
2. Feet are together (or up to 6 inches apart), toes and balls of the feet touching the floor
3. The starting position requires that your elbows be bent, chest be one inch off the floor, and body be perfectly straight from head-to-ankles

Execution

1. Shift your body weight (without moving your hands or feet) so your right chest is by your right hand
2. As you push away from the floor, use your right arm for the majority of the pushing, using your left only for assistance, extend your arms, and exhale as you reach the top
   a. keep your elbows near your ribs (either touching your sides or up to just a few inches away) as this is a more functional way of applying a pushing motion
   b. keep your body in a straight line from head-to-ankles
   c. exhale as you push away from the floor
3. When you reach the top, begin to lower yourself towards the floor with most of your weight over your right arm, inhale
4. Stop when the right side of your chest touches your right hand
5. Shift your body weight so your left chest is by your left hand and repeat the motion over on your left side (when you have done a repetition once on the right and once on the left, this is considered just ONE complete repetition)
6. Repeat for a desired amount of repetitions per set

Body Parts Involved

This exercise works the same muscle groups as the standard 4 – point push up (chest – pectoral muscles, front of shoulder – anterior deltoid muscle, back of the upper arms - triceps) except that greater demands are placed on the side you happen to be leaning on. The body shifting from right to left and vice versa while the chest is one inch away from the floor also seems to produce more soreness in the pectoral muscles, meaning greater conditioning gains will take place in the chest area.

Note: To place more of your bodyweight over your arms, you may elevate both feet by placing them on steps of progressively increasing height, a chair, or couch. This effectively increases the weight you must push off the floor resulting in greater strength and muscle mass gains when utilized with the appropriate repetitions per set scheme.

Side-to-Side, Bottom Starting, 4 – Point Push Ups

1

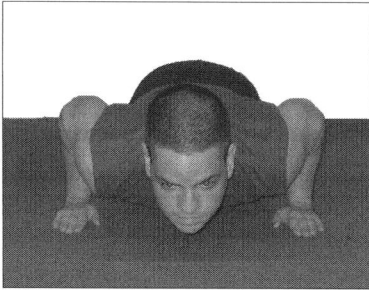

2

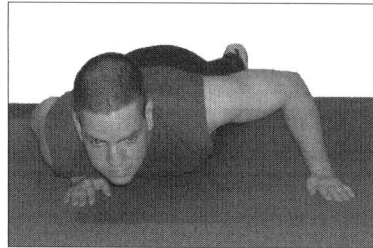

3

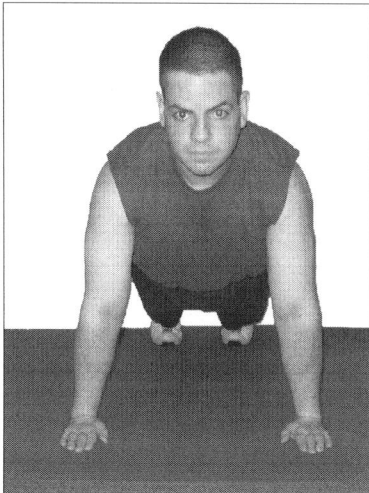

4

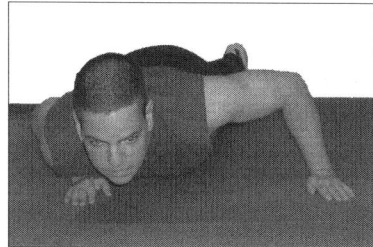

5

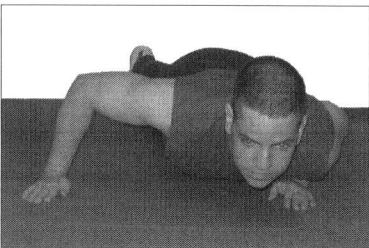

6

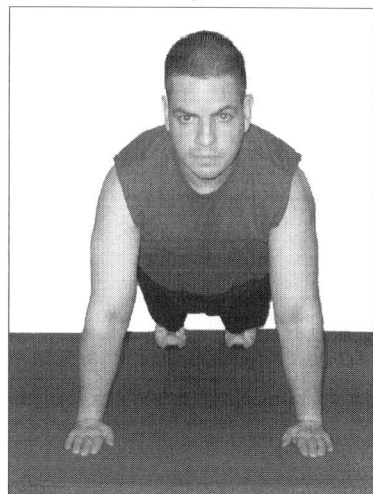

One – Arm, Assisted, 3 – Point Push Ups

Starting Position

1. Begin with your right hand flat on the floor, at chest level, in line with the right side of your chest
2. Feet are spread out about 2 shoulder widths apart, toes and balls of the feet touching the floor
3. The starting position requires that your right arm be extended, and that your left arm be bent with your left hand hovering somewhere between the floor and your left chest area
4. The body should be perfectly straight from head-to-ankles

Execution

1. Lower yourself towards the floor with your right arm, allowing the thumb, index finger, and middle finger of the left hand to press against the floor for assistance as needed
2. Inhale on the way down, keep your elbow near your right side, maintain a straight body from head-to-ankles
3. Stop when your chin is within one inch from the floor
4. As you push away from the floor with your right arm, allow the thumb, index finger, and middle finger of the left hand to push away from the floor for assistance as needed
5. Exhale as you return to the starting position
6. Repeat for a desired amount of repetitions per set
7. Repeat with left arm

Body Parts Involved

This exercise works the same muscle groups as the standard 4 – point push up (chest – pectoral muscles, front of shoulder – anterior deltoid muscle, back of the upper arms - triceps) except that greater demands are placed on the side you are emphasizing than any other previous push up exercise.

Note: To place more of your bodyweight over your arms, you may elevate both feet by placing them on steps of progressively increasing height, a chair, or couch. This effectively increases the weight you must push off the floor resulting in greater strength and muscle mass gains when utilized with the appropriate repetitions per set scheme.

One – Arm, Assisted, 3 – Point Push Ups

1

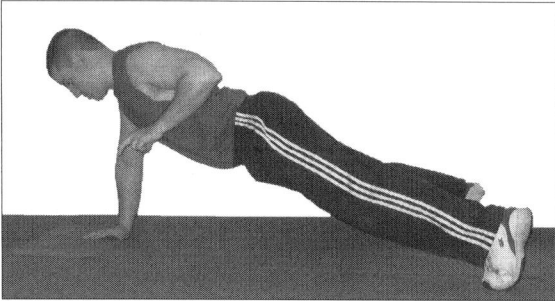

1a

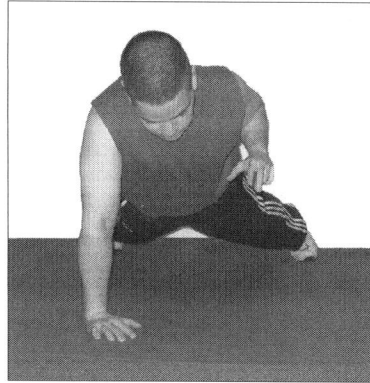

2

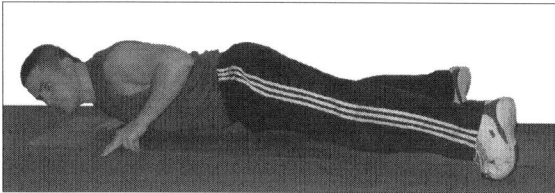

2a

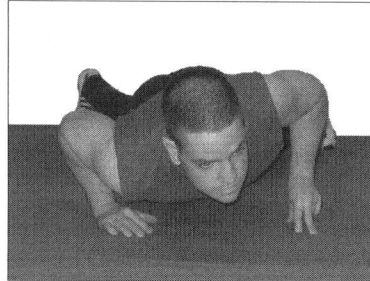

3

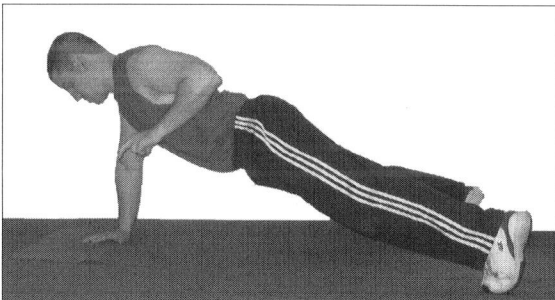

3a

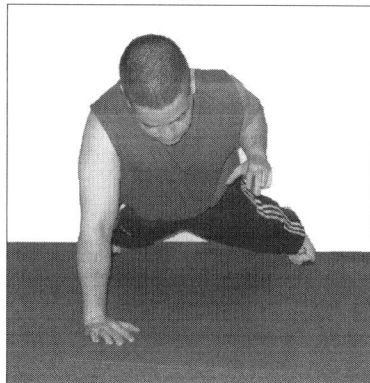

One – Arm, 3 – Point Push Ups

Starting Position

1. Begin with your right hand flat on the floor, at chest level, in line with the right side of your chest
2. Feet are spread out about 2 shoulder widths apart, toes and balls of the feet touching the floor
3. The starting position requires that your right arm be extended, and that your left arm be placed behind your back
4. The body should be perfectly straight from head-to-ankles

Execution

1. Lower yourself towards the floor with your right arm
2. Inhale on the way down, keep your elbow near your right side, maintain a straight body from head-to-ankles
3. Stop when your chin is within one inch from the floor
4. Push away from the floor with your right arm
5. Exhale as you return to the starting position
6. Repeat for a desired amount of repetitions per set
7. Repeat with left arm

Body Parts Involved

This exercise works the same muscle groups as the standard 4 – point push up (chest – pectoral muscles, front of shoulder – anterior deltoid muscle, back of the upper arms - triceps) except that greater demands are placed on the side you are emphasizing than any other previous push up exercise.

Note: To place more of your bodyweight over your arms, you may elevate both feet by placing them on steps of progressively increasing height, a chair, or couch. This effectively increases the weight you must push off the floor resulting in greater strength and muscle mass gains when utilized with the appropriate repetitions per set scheme.

One – Arm, 3 – Point Push Ups

1

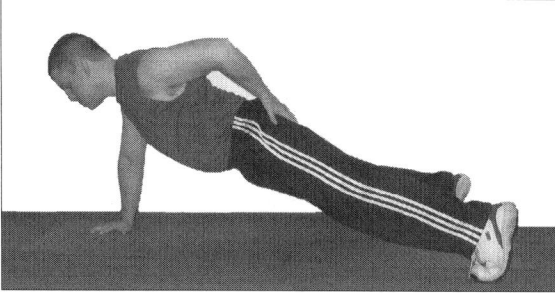

1a

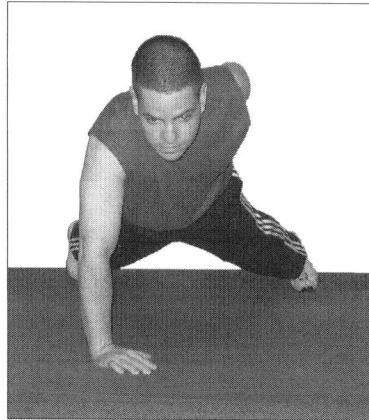

2

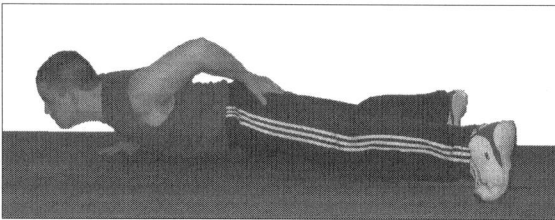

2a

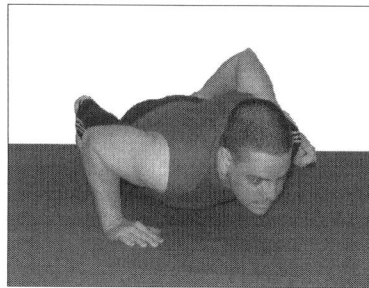

3

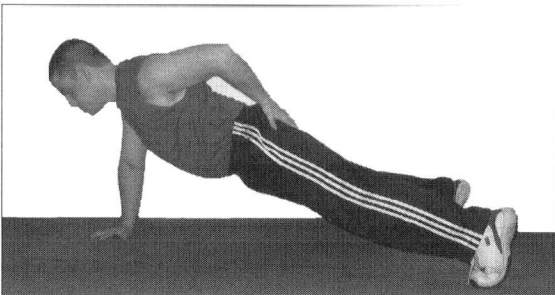

3a

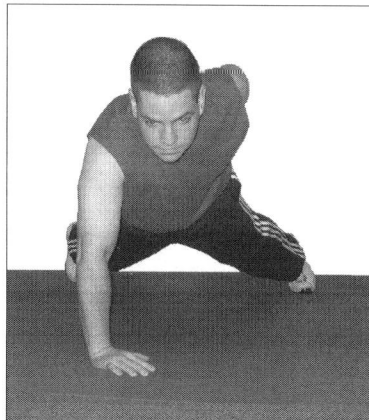

One – Arm, 2 – Point Push Ups
(1 hand and opposite foot touching floor)

Starting Position

1. Begin with your right arm extended, hand flat on the floor at chest level, in line with the right side of your chest
2. Your left arm can be placed behind your back or extended out, elevated off the floor as if in a Superman flying position (to aid with balance)
3. Feet are spread out about 1 ½ shoulder widths apart with the toes and balls of the left foot touching the floor and the right foot elevated off the ground
4. The body should be perfectly straight from head-to-ankle

Execution

1. Lower yourself towards the floor with your right arm
2. Inhale on the way down, keep your elbow near your right side, maintain a straight body from head-to-ankles
3. Stop when your chin is within one inch from the floor
4. Push away from the floor with your right arm
5. Exhale as you return to the starting position
6. Repeat for a desired amount of repetitions per set
7. Repeat with left hand and right foot touching the floor

Body Parts Involved

This exercise works the same muscle groups as the standard 4 – point push up (chest – pectoral muscles, front of shoulder – anterior deltoid muscle, back of the upper arms - triceps) except that greater demands are placed on the side you are emphasizing. Your abdominal muscles are also being used more as they are stressed to stabilize your body and keep your back straight.

Note: To place more of your bodyweight over your arms, you may elevate your feet by placing them on steps of progressively increasing height, a chair, or couch. This effectively increases the weight you must push off the floor resulting in greater strength and muscle mass gains when utilized with the appropriate repetitions per set scheme.

One – Arm, 2 – Point Push Ups
(1 hand and opposite foot touching floor)

1

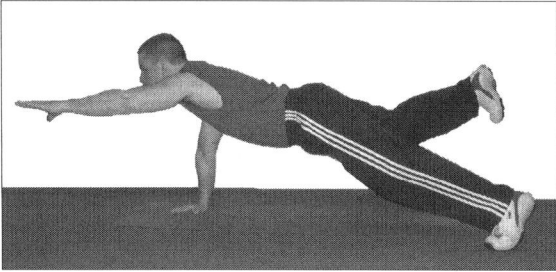

1a

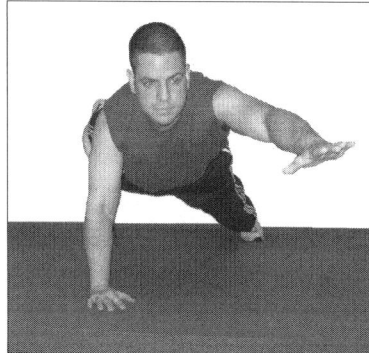

2

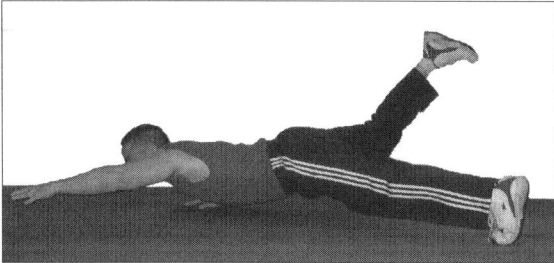

2a

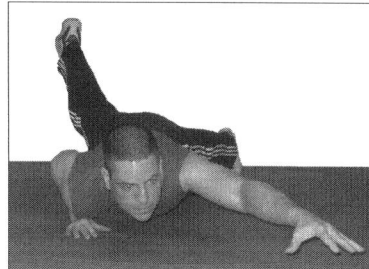

3

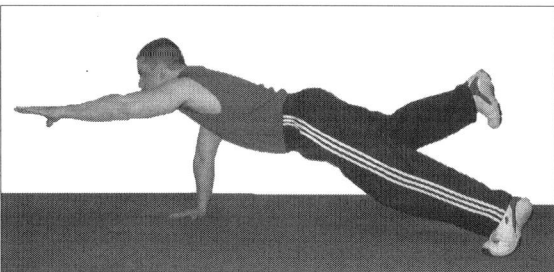

3a

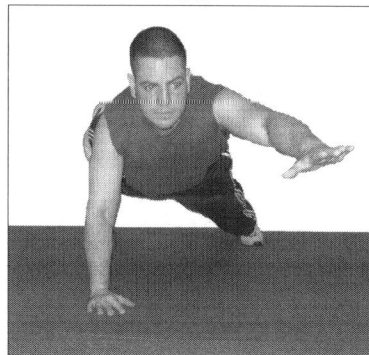

2 – Point Push Ups
(Both hands touching the floor, no feet touching the floor)

Starting Position

1. Assume a tuck planche position by:
   a. dropping into a full squat and placing your hands on the ground, in front of your feet
   b. rest your knees to the outside of your elbows
   c. lean forward until your feet are off the floor and your weight is on your hands
   d. knees are resting on your elbows supporting some of your weight
   e. continue to raise the hips until they are slightly higher than your shoulders
   f. knees will move off the elbows and to the rear
   g. straighten both arms
2. Back is straight and angled slightly downward from hips (higher) to shoulders (lower)
3. Shoulders will be more forward than the hands
4. Arms are straight and extended

Execution

1. Lower yourself towards the floor keeping several tips in mind:
   a. keep your elbows near your ribs (either touching your sides or up to just a few inches away) as this is a more functional way of applying a pushing motion
   b. keep your body in a straight line from shoulder-to-hips
   c. inhale as you lower yourself
2. Stop when your knees and chin are within one inch of the floor
3. As you push away from the floor, extend your arms, exhale, and return to the starting position
4. Repeat for a desired amount of repetitions per set

Body Parts Involved

This exercise will work the muscle groups:
1. chest (pectoral muscles)
2. front of the shoulder (anterior deltoid muscle)
3. back of the upper arms (triceps)
Also highly worked muscle groups include:
1. upper and middle back (trapezius and rhomboids)
2. sides of your back (latissimus dorsi)
3. Abdominal muscles

Note: To create a greater range of motion, and allow you to lower yourself without knees touching the ground, you can support yourself between two chairs.

2 – Point Push Ups
(Both hands touching the floor, no feet touching the floor)

1

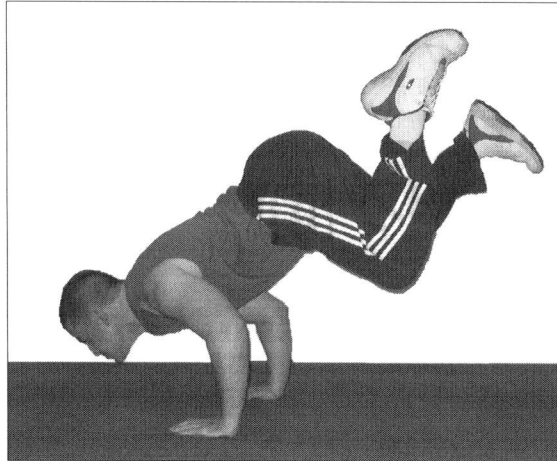

2

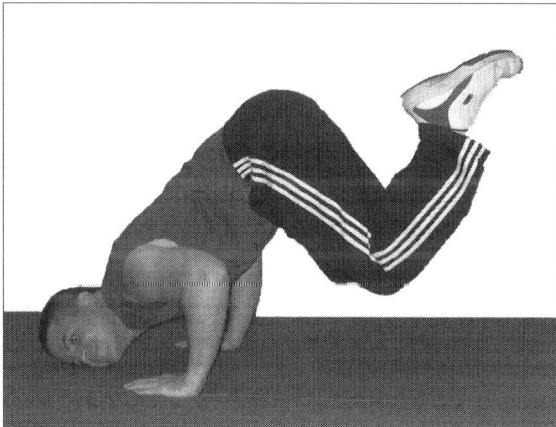

3

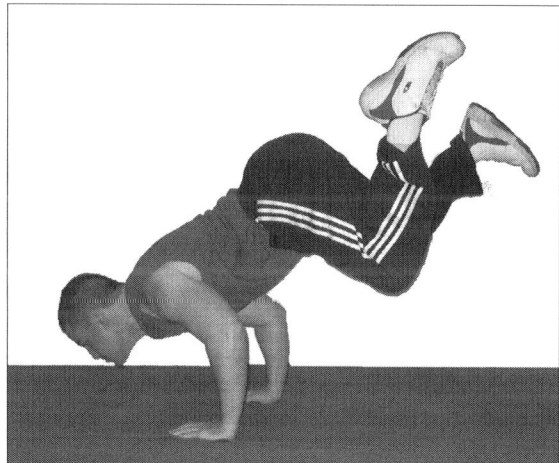

Power Push Ups

Modified Hand Stand Push Ups

Starting Position

1. Elevate both feet onto a chair or couch so they are about shoulder width apart
2. Your hands are on the floor in standard push up position about shoulder width apart or more
3. While keeping your legs as straight as possible, and without moving your feet, begin to crawl backwards with your hands, bending at the hips
4. Your upper body and legs should form an "L" shape and be bent close to a 90 degree angle at the hips, with your upper body in a near vertical position
5. Extend your arms so they are straight and head is off the floor

Execution

1. Lower yourself towards the floor (while inhaling) until your head touches the floor
2. Elbows will be to the sides and away from your body
3. While exhaling, push yourself away from the floor until your arms are straight and extended, returning to the starting position
4. Repeat for a desired amount of repetitions per set

Body Parts Involved

1. Shoulder (deltoids)
2. Upper back (upper trapezius)
3. Back of the upper arms (triceps)
4. Minor involvement of the upper chest (pectorals)

Modified Hand Stand Push Ups

1

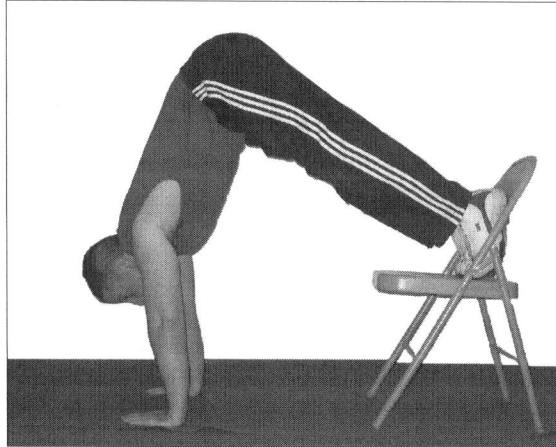

2

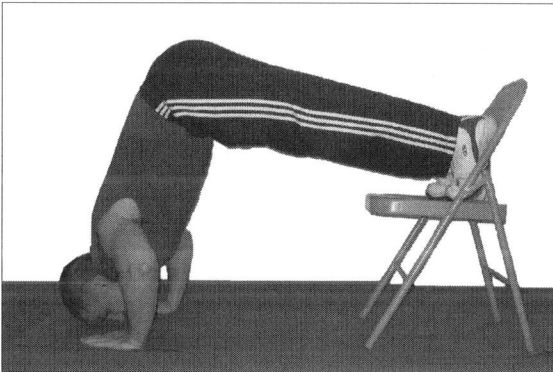

3

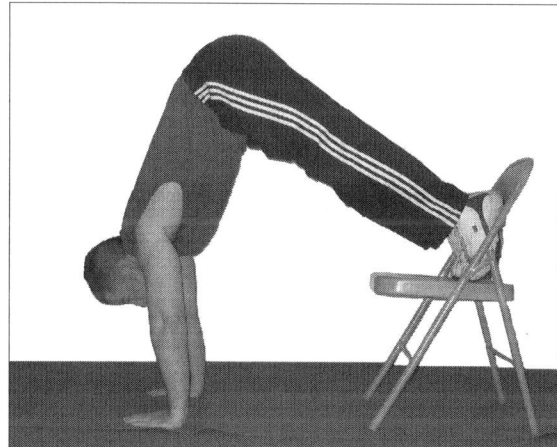

Hand Stand Push Ups

Starting Position

1. Dropping into a full squat (in front of a wall), place your hands flat on the floor, in front of your feet, and shoulder width apart (about 8 inches from the wall)
2. Push off with your feet until you are upside down with your back towards the wall, legs straight up and heels touching the wall
3. Arms are extended and straight

Execution

1. Lower yourself towards the floor (while inhaling) until your head touches the floor
2. Elbows will be to the sides and away from your body
3. While exhaling, push yourself away from the floor until your arms are straight and extended, returning to the starting position
4. Repeat for a desired amount of repetitions per set

Body Parts Involved

1. Shoulder (deltoids)
2. Upper back (upper trapezius)
3. Back of the upper arms (triceps)
4. Minor involvement of the upper chest (pectorals)

Note: To increase the range of motion, you can place your hands on two chairs, lowering yourself between them.

Hand Stand Push Ups

1

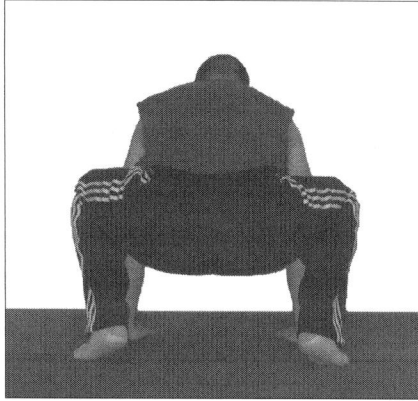

2

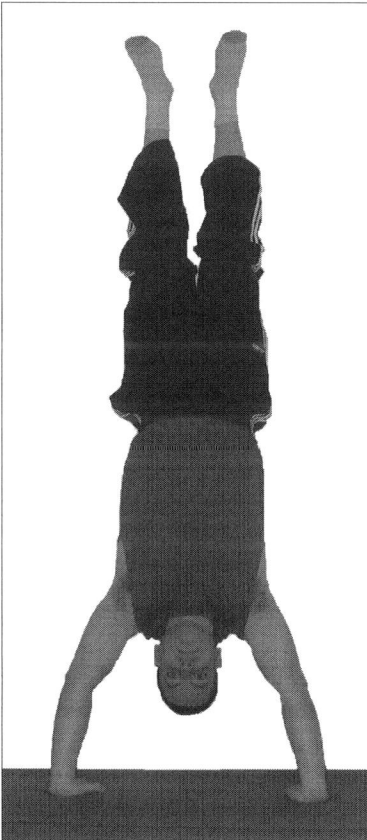

3

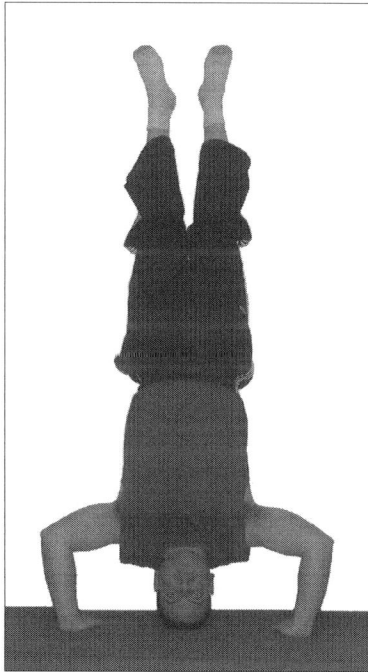

4

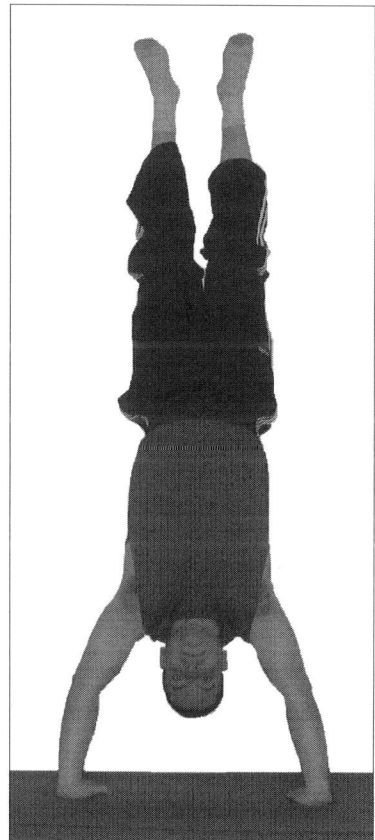

Side-to-Side, Top Starting, Hand Stand Push Ups

Starting Position

1. Dropping into a full squat (in front of a wall), place your hands flat on the floor, in front of your feet, and shoulder width apart (about 8 inches from the wall)
2. Push off with your feet until you are upside down with your back towards the wall, legs straight up and heels touching the wall
3. Arms are extended and straight

Execution

1. Shift your body weight (without moving your hands) so it is over your right arm
2. Lower yourself towards the floor (while inhaling) with most of your weight over your right arm until your head touches the floor
3. Elbows will be to the sides and away from your body
4. As you push away from the floor, use your right arm for the majority of the pushing, using your left only for assistance, extend your arms, exhale, return to the top starting position
5. Shift your body weight so it is over your left arm and repeat the motion over your left side (when you have done a repetition once on the right and once on the left, this is considered just ONE complete repetition)
6. Repeat for a desired amount of repetitions per set

Body Parts Involved

Greater emphasis is placed on the side you happen to be leaning on.

1. Shoulder (deltoids)
2. Upper back (upper trapezius)
3. Back of the upper arms (triceps)
4. Minor involvement of the upper chest (pectorals)

Side-to-Side, Top Starting, Hand Stand Push Ups

1

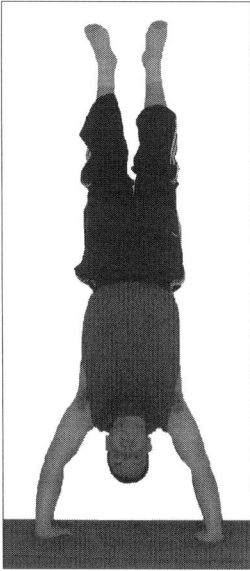

2

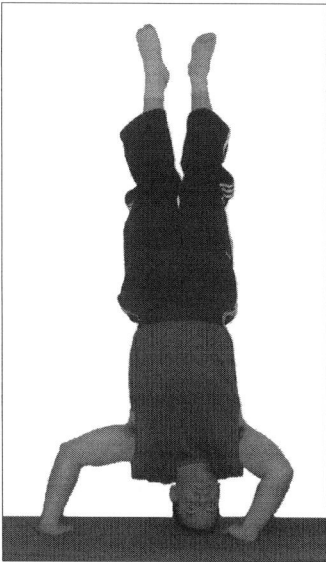

3

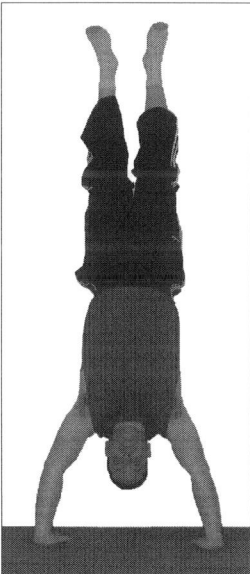

4

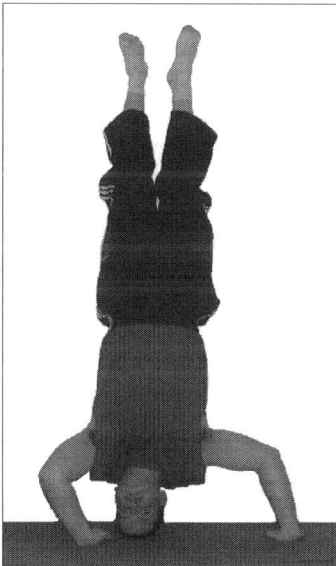

5

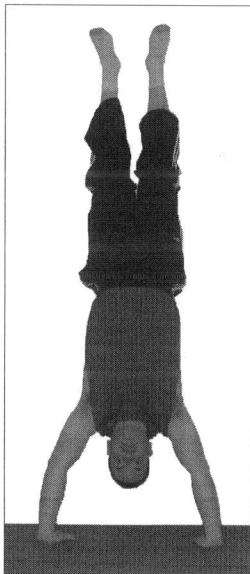

Side-to-Side, Bottom Starting, Hand Stand Push Ups

Starting Position

1. Dropping into a full squat (in front of a wall), place your hands flat on the floor, in front of your feet, and shoulder width apart (about 8 inches from the wall)
2. Push off with your feet until you are upside down with your back towards the wall, legs straight up and heels touching the wall
3. Arms are bent, with head touching the floor

Execution

1. Shift your body weight (without moving your hands) so it is on your right side
2. As you push away from the floor, use your right arm for the majority of the pushing, using your left only for assistance, extend your arms, exhale
3. During the push, elbows will be to the sides and away from your body
4. Now, lower yourself towards the floor (while inhaling) with most of your weight over your right arm until your head touches the floor, returning to the bottom starting position
5. Shift your body weight so it is on your left side and repeat the motion over your left side (when you have done a repetition once on the right and once on the left, this is considered just ONE complete repetition)
6. Repeat for a desired amount of repetitions per set

Body Parts Involved

Greater emphasis is placed on the side you happen to be leaning on.

1. Shoulder (deltoids)
2. Upper back (upper trapezius)
3. Back of the upper arms (triceps)
4. Minor involvement of the upper chest (pectorals)

Side-to-Side, Bottom Starting, Hand Stand Push Ups

1
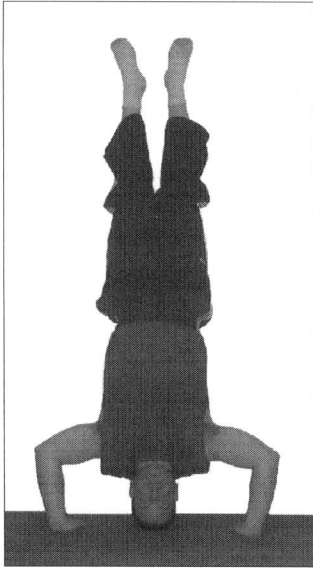

2
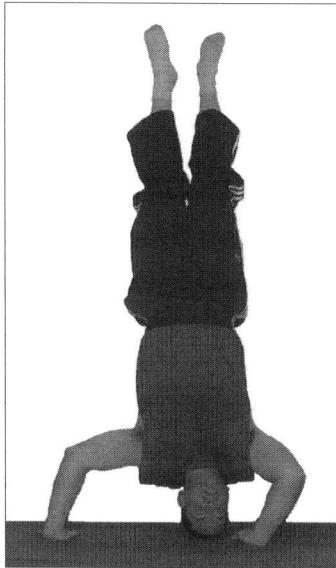

3
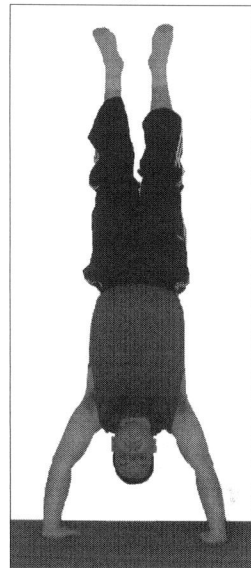

4
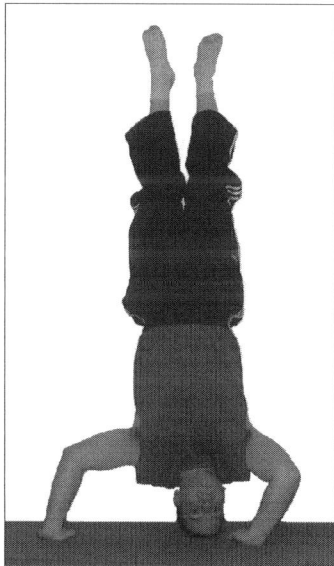

5
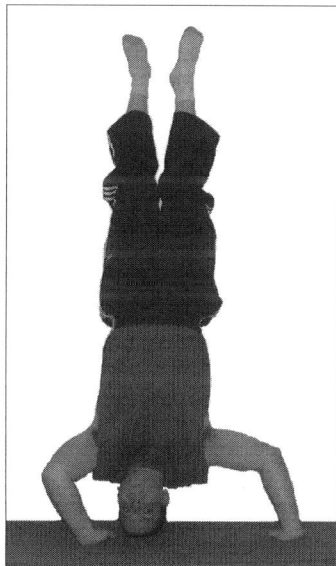

6
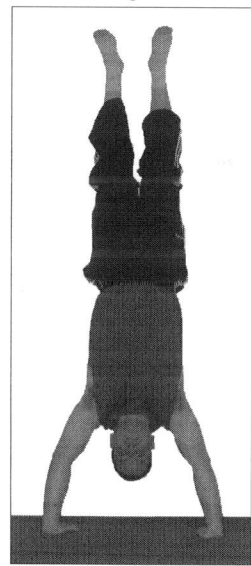

Reverse 4 – Point Push Ups

Starting Position

1. Lay flat on your back
2. Bend both knees until your heels are very close to and under your buttocks
3. At this point, your hips and buttocks should be off the floor, your heels are off the floor and balls of your feet are flat on the floor
4. Place both hands flat on the floor somewhere between your shoulders and ears
5. Your elbows should be pointing straight up with arms bent, palms flat on the floor, and finger tips pointing towards your feet
6. Points touching the floor should be balls of the feet, shoulders, palms of the hands, and head

Execution

1. Push yourself off the floor extending your arms to straighten them as much as possible
2. At the same time, your hips should push upward, your back will arch, and your legs will also push against the floor (all this while exhaling)
3. The top position should be a complete back-bridge with top of the head pointing towards the floor
4. As you inhale, lower yourself until your shoulders, neck and head touch the floor
5. Repeat for a desired amount of repetitions per set

Body Parts Involved

1. Back of the upper arms (triceps)
2. Upper back (trapezius)
3. Middle back (rhomboids)
4. Lower back (sacrospinalis)

Reverse 4 – Point Push Ups

1

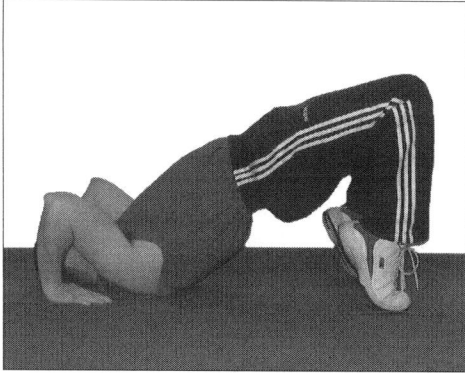

1a

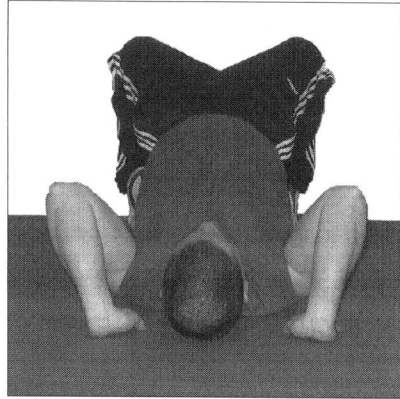

2

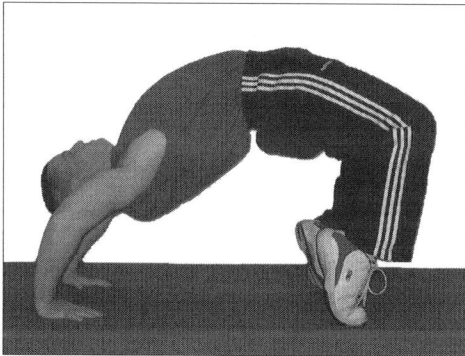

2a

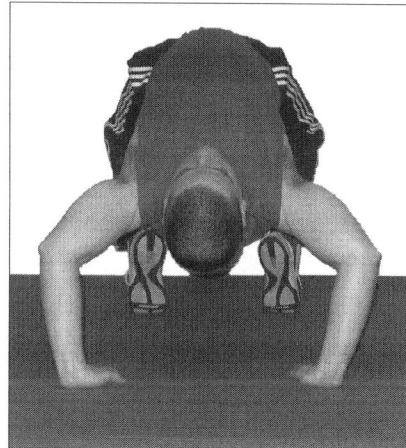

3

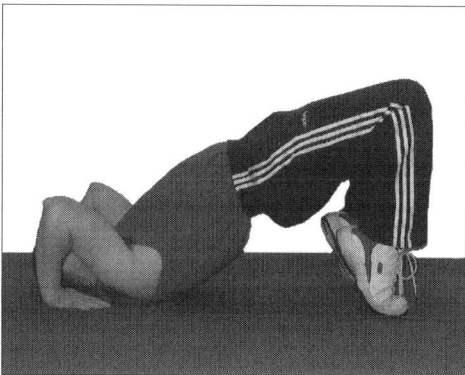

3a

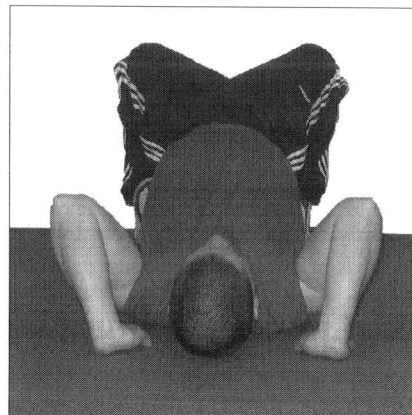

Side-to-Side, Top Starting, Reverse Push Ups

Starting Position

1. Lay flat on your back
2. Bend both knees until your heels are very close to and under your buttocks
3. At this point, your hips and buttocks should be off the floor, your heels are off the floor and balls of your feet are flat on the floor
4. Place both hands flat on the floor somewhere between your shoulders and ears
5. Your elbows should be pointing straight up with arms bent, palms flat on the floor, and finger tips pointing towards your feet
6. Points touching the floor should be balls of the feet, shoulders, palms of the hands, and head
7. Push yourself off the floor extending your arms to straighten them as much as possible creating a complete back-bridge with the top of the head pointing towards the floor

Execution

1. Shift your body weight (without moving your hands) so it is over your right arm
2. Lower yourself towards the floor (while inhaling) with most of your weight over your right arm until your shoulders, neck and head touch the floor
3. As you push away from the floor, use your right arm for the majority of the pushing, using your left only for assistance, extend your arms, exhale, return to the top starting position
4. Shift your body weight so it is over your left arm and repeat the motion over your left side (when you have done a repetition once on the right and once on the left, this is considered just ONE complete repetition)
5. Repeat for a desired amount of repetitions per set

Body Parts Involved

Greater emphasis is placed on the side you happen to be leaning on.

1. Back of the upper arms (triceps)
2. Upper back (trapezius)
3. Middle back (rhomboids)
4. Lower back (sacrospinalis)

Side-to-Side, Top Starting, Reverse Push Ups

1

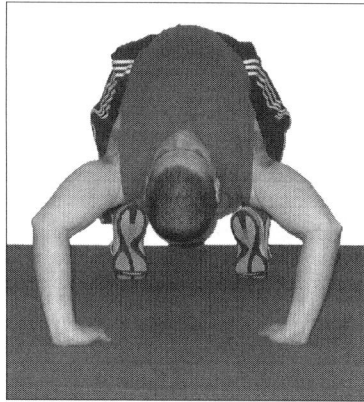

2

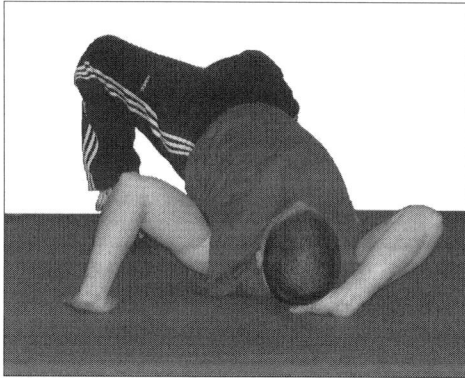

3

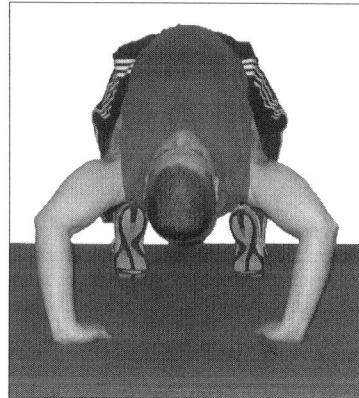

4

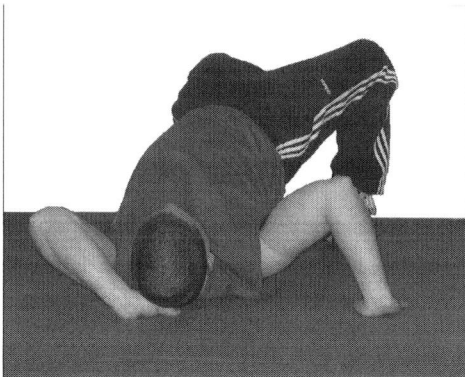

5

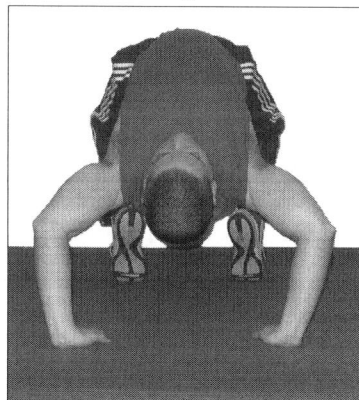

Side-to-Side, Bottom Starting, Reverse Push Ups

Starting Position

1. Lay flat on your back
2. Bend both knees until your heels are very close to and under your buttocks
3. At this point, your hips and buttocks should be off the floor, your heels are off the floor and balls of your feet are flat on the floor
4. Place both hands flat on the floor somewhere between your shoulders and ears
5. Your elbows should be pointing straight up with arms bent, palms flat on the floor, and finger tips pointing towards your feet
6. Points touching the floor should be balls of the feet, shoulders, palms of the hands, and head

Execution

1. Shift your body weight (without moving your hands) so it is by your right side
2. As you push away from the floor, use your right arm for the majority of the pushing, using your left only for assistance, extend your arms as much as possible while exhaling
3. At the same time, your hips should push upward, your back will arch, and your legs will also push against the floor
4. The top position should be a complete back-bridge with top of the head pointing towards the floor
5. Lower yourself towards the floor (while inhaling) with most of your weight over your right arm until your shoulders, neck and head touch the floor
6. Shift your body weight so it is by your left arm and repeat the motion over your left side (when you have done a repetition once on the right and once on the left, this is considered just ONE complete repetition)
7. Repeat for a desired amount of repetitions per set

Body Parts Involved

Greater emphasis is placed on the side you happen to be leaning on.

1. Back of the upper arms (triceps)
2. Upper back (trapezius)
3. Middle back (rhomboids)
4. Lower back (sacrospinalis)

Side-to-Side, Bottom Starting, Reverse Push Ups

1

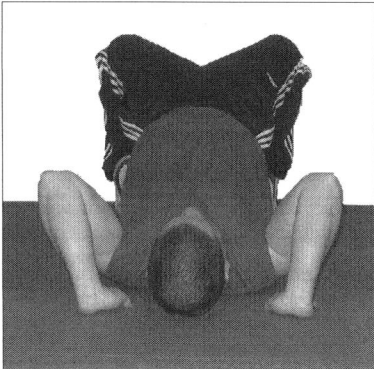

2

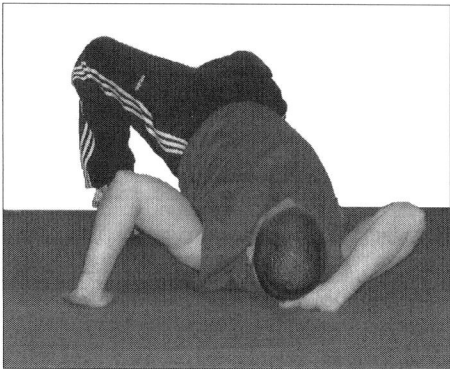

3

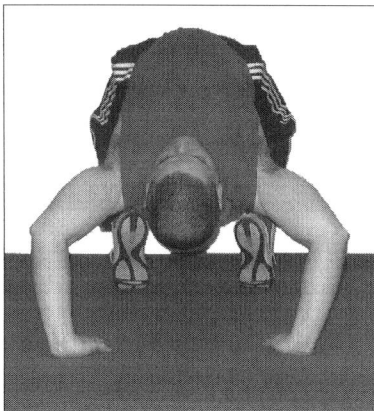

4

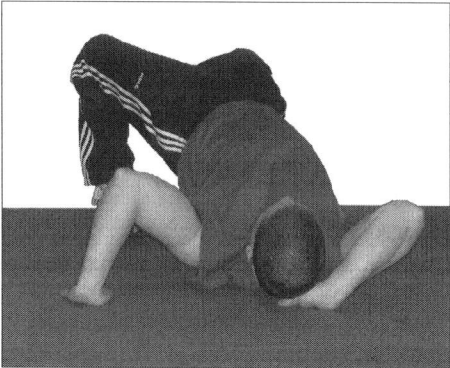

5

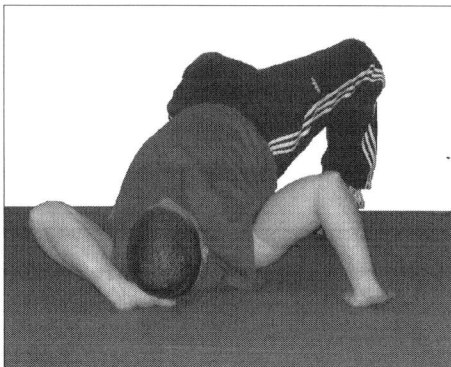

6

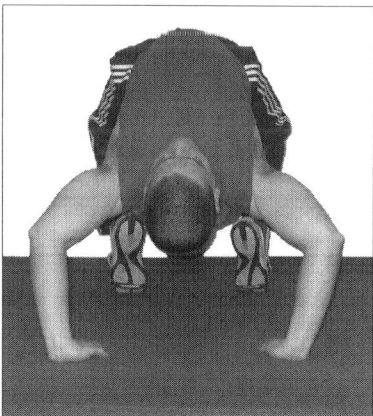

One – Arm, Reverse, 3 – Point Push Ups

Starting Position

1. Lay flat on your back
2. Bend both knees until your heels are very close to and under your buttocks
3. At this point, your hips and buttocks should be off the floor, your heels are off the floor and balls of your feet are flat on the floor
4. Place your right hand flat on the floor somewhere between your shoulders and ears
5. Left hand can be placed along side the left hip
6. Your right elbow should be pointing straight up with your arm bent, palm flat on the floor, and finger tips pointing towards your feet
7. Points touching the floor should be balls of the feet, shoulders, palm of your right hand, and head

Execution

1. Push yourself off the floor extending your arm to straighten it as much as possible
2. At the same time, your hips should push upward, your back will arch, and your legs will also push against the floor (all this while exhaling)
3. The top position should be a complete back-bridge with top of the head pointing towards the floor
4. As you inhale, lower yourself until your shoulders, neck and head touch the floor
5. Repeat for a desired amount of repetitions per set
6. Repeat with the left arm

Body Parts Involved

All the emphasis is placed on the side you are using more than any other reverse push up variation.

1. Back of the upper arms (triceps)
2. Upper back (trapezius)
3. Middle back (rhomboids)
4. Lower back (sacrospinalis)

One – Arm, Reverse, 3 – Point Push Ups

1

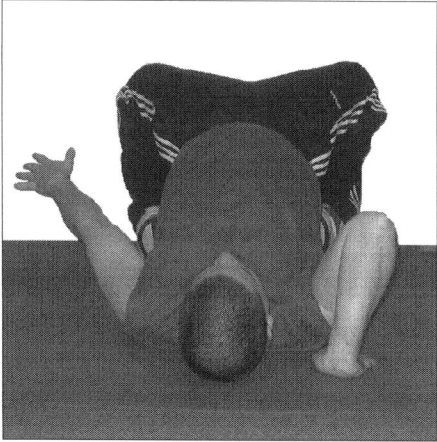

2

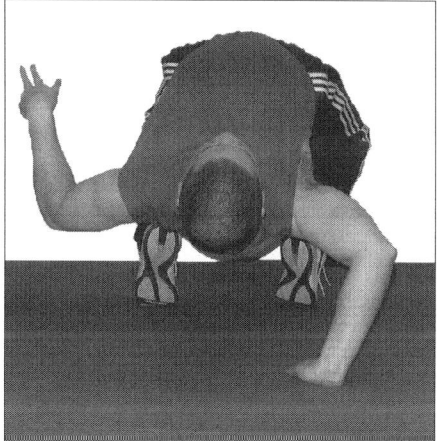

3

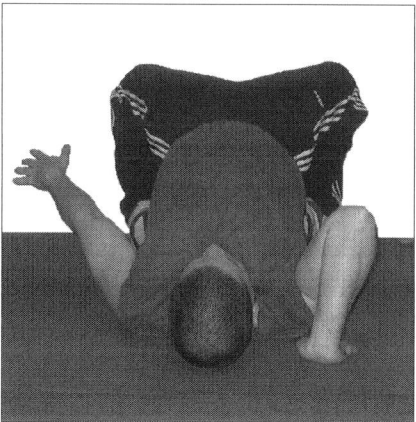

Dipping Strength

Standard 4 – Point Dips

Starting Position

1. Place two chairs facing each other about 3 to 4 feet apart.
2. Sit on one chair, facing the other with your hands supporting your weight by grabbing the left and right corners of the chair, fingers facing forward
3. Lift your feet and place them on the other chair, moving your body slightly forward so it is suspended between the two chairs
4. Arms are extended and straight

Execution

1. While inhaling, begin to lower yourself towards the floor until your elbows bend 90 degrees
2. Arms should be parallel to each other with elbows in tight
3. Torso can be straight up and down
4. As you push away from the floor, exhale, extend your arms, and return to the starting position
5. Repeat for a desired amount of repetitions per set

Body Parts Involved

1. Back of the upper arms (triceps)
2. Back of the shoulders (posterior deltoids)
3. If your body is straight up and down, some chest (pectorals) and some upper back (trapezius)
4. If your body is leaning forward, then more chest (pectorals)
5. If your body is leaning back, then more upper back (trapezius)

Standard 4 – Point Dips

1

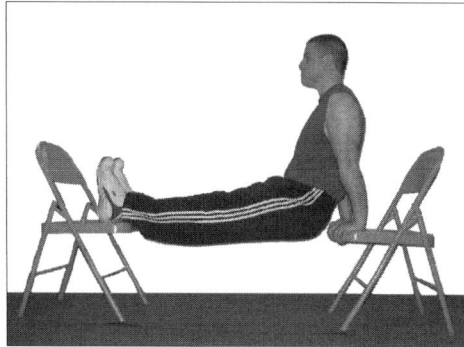

2

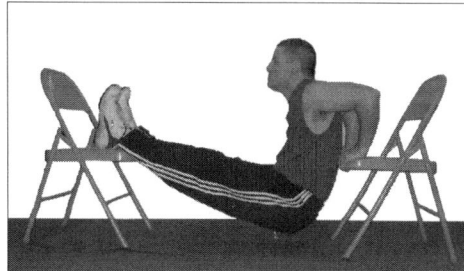

3

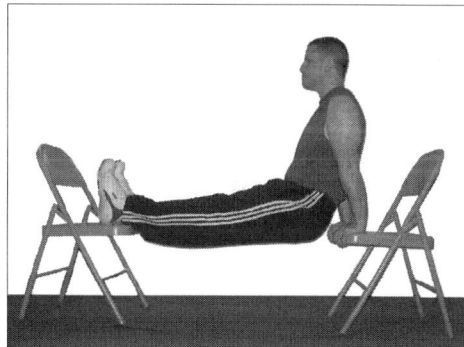

Side-to-Side, Top Starting, 4 – Point Dips

Starting Position

1. Place two chairs facing each other to the left and right of you, and a third chair about 3 to 4 feet in front of you
2. Face the third chair while your hands support your weight by placing them on the left and right chairs, fingers facing forward
3. Lift your feet and place them on the third chair, moving your body slightly forward so it is suspended between all three chairs
4. Arms are extended and straight

Execution

1. Shift your body weight (without moving your hands) so it is over your right arm
2. Lower yourself towards the floor (while inhaling) with most of your weight over your right arm until your right elbow bends 90 degrees
3. Torso can be straight up and down with elbows close to your body
4. As you push away from the floor, use your right arm for the majority of the pushing, using your left only for assistance, extend your arms, exhale, return to the top starting position
5. Shift your body weight so it is over your left arm and repeat the motion over your left side (when you have done a repetition once on the right and once on the left, this is considered just ONE complete repetition)
6. Repeat for a desired amount of repetitions per set

Body Parts Involved

Greater emphasis is placed on the side you happen to be leaning on.

1. Back of the upper arms (triceps)
2. Back of the shoulders (posterior deltoids)
3. If your body is straight up and down, some chest (pectorals) and some upper back (trapezius)
4. If your body is leaning forward, then more chest (pectorals)
5. If your body is leaning back, then more upper back (trapezius)

Side-to-Side, Top Starting, 4 – Point Dips

1

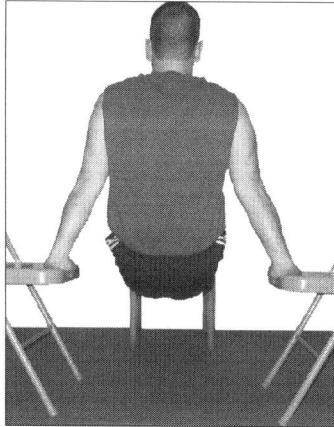

2

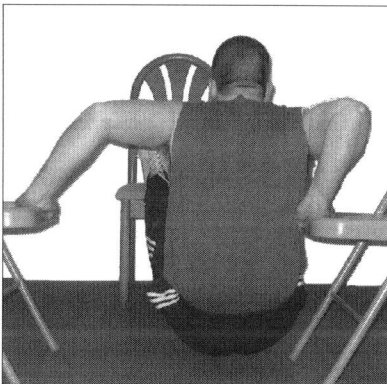

3

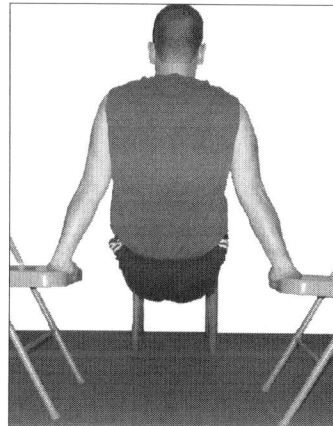

4

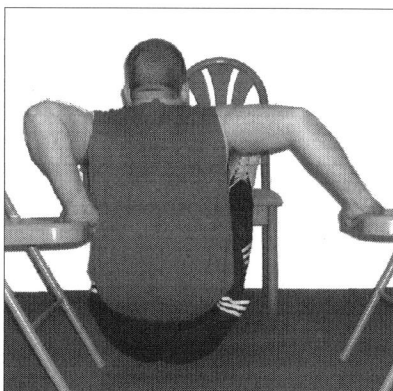

5

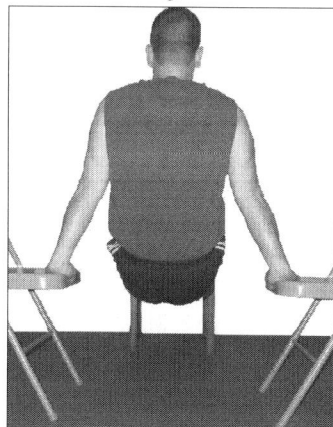

Side-to-Side, Bottom Starting, 4 – Point Dips

Starting Position

1. Place two chairs facing each other to the left and right of you, and a third chair about 3 to 4 feet in front of you
2. Face the third chair while your hands support your weight by placing them on the left and right chairs, fingers facing forward
3. Lift your feet and place them on the third chair, moving your body slightly forward so it is suspended between all three chairs
4. Arms are bent so the elbows are at a 90 degree angle

Execution

1. Shift your body weight (without moving your hands) so it is by your right arm
2. As you push away from the floor, use your right arm for the majority of the pushing, using your left only for assistance, extend your arms and exhale
3. Now lower yourself towards the floor (while inhaling) with most of your weight over your right arm until your right elbow bends 90 degrees
4. Shift your body weight so it is by your left arm and repeat the motion over your left side (when you have done a repetition once on the right and once on the left, this is considered just ONE complete repetition)
5. Repeat for a desired amount of repetitions per set

Body Parts Involved

Greater emphasis is placed on the side you happen to be leaning on.

1. Back of the upper arms (triceps)
2. Back of the shoulders (posterior deltoids)
3. If your body is straight up and down, some chest (pectorals) and some upper back (trapezius)
4. If your body is leaning forward, then more chest (pectorals)
5. If your body is leaning back, then more upper back (trapezius)

Side-to-Side, Bottom Starting, 4 – Point Dips

1

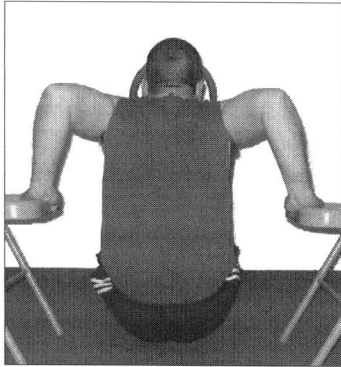

2

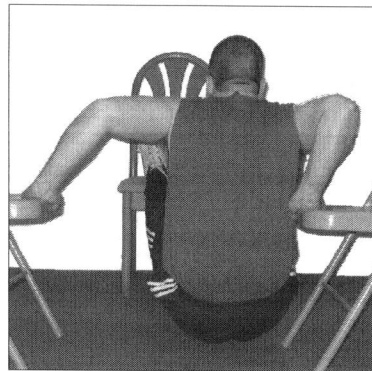

3

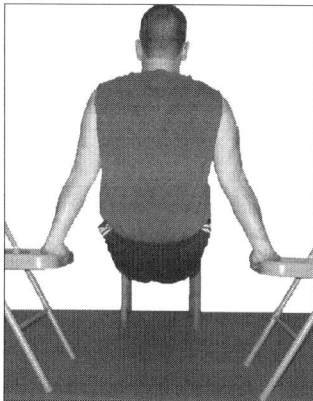

4

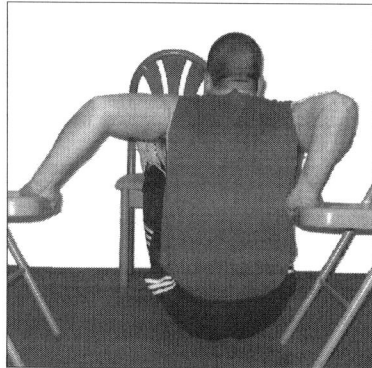

5

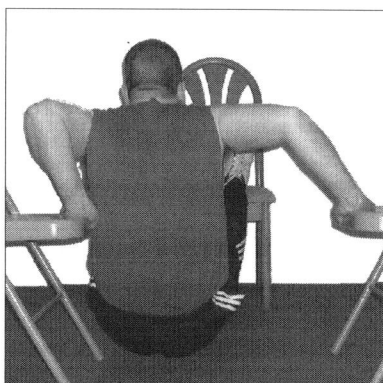

6

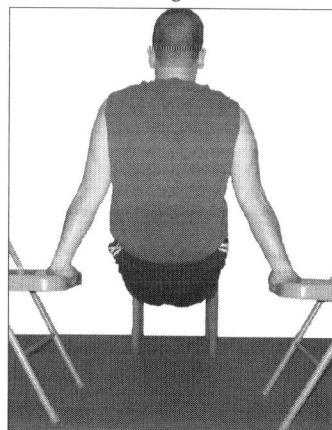

One – Arm, 3 – Point Dips

Starting Position

1. Using a chair, place your right hand on the seat, supporting your weight
2. Arm is extended, left hand can be placed on your left hip
3. Facing your feet, place them flat on the ground about 3 feet from the chair and 1 ½ to 2 shoulder widths apart

Execution

1. While inhaling, begin to lower yourself towards the floor until your right elbow is bent 90 degrees
2. Elbow should be close to your body
3. Torso can be straight up and down
4. As you push away from the floor, exhale, extend your arm, and return to the starting position
5. Repeat for a desired amount of repetitions per set
6. Repeat with the left arm

Body Parts Involved

All the emphasis is placed on the side you are working on.

1. Back of the upper arms (triceps)
2. Back of the shoulders (posterior deltoids)
3. If your body is straight up and down, some chest (pectorals) and some upper back (trapezius)
4. If your body is leaning forward, then more chest (pectorals)
5. If your body is leaning back, then more upper back (trapezius)

Note: More advanced people can place their feet on 2 chairs spaced 1 ½ to 2 shoulder widths apart for even greater strength and muscle gains.

One – Arm, 3 – Point Dips

1

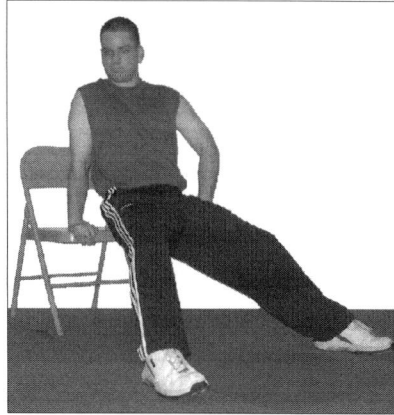

2

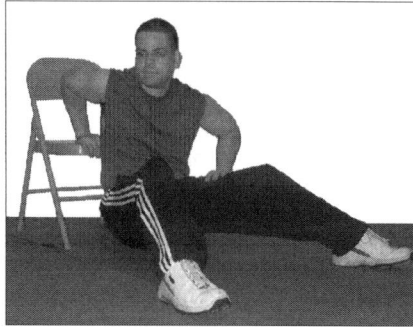

3

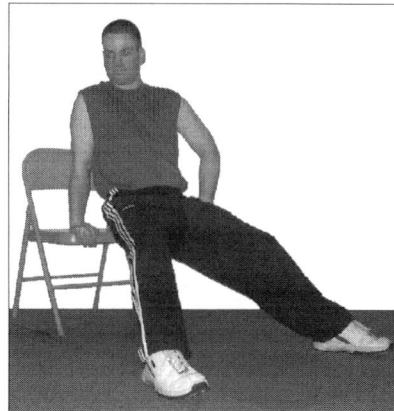

2 – Point Dips
(Supported by both hands; feet and legs are suspended)

Starting Position

1. Place two chairs next to you (one on the left and one on the right)
2. With your arms extended and straight, place the palms of each hand respectively on the left and right chair
3. Support your full weight by lifting your legs and feet off the floor so your legs are straight and parallel to the floor

Execution

1. While inhaling, begin to lower yourself towards the floor until your elbows bend 90 degrees
2. Arms should be parallel to each other with elbows in tight
3. Legs remain straight and parallel to the floor
4. Torso can be straight up and down
5. As you push away from the floor, exhale, extend your arms, and return to the starting position
6. Repeat for a desired amount of repetitions per set

Body Parts Involved

1. Back of the upper arms (triceps)
2. Back of the shoulders (posterior deltoids)
3. Stomach area (abdominals)
4. If your body is straight up and down, some chest (pectorals) and some upper back (trapezius)
5. If your body is leaning forward, then more chest (pectorals)
6. If your body is leaning back, then more upper back (trapezius)

2 – Point Dips
(Supported by both hands; feet and legs are suspended)

1

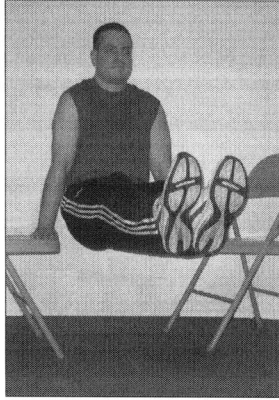

2

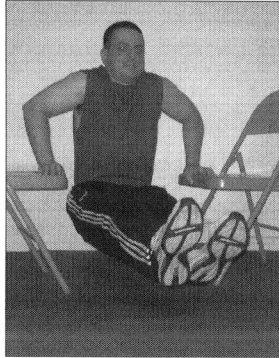

3

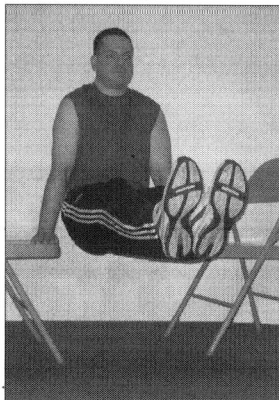

Side-to-Side, Top Starting, 2 – Point Dips
(Supported by both hands; feet and legs are suspended)

Starting Position

1. Place two chairs next to you (one on the left and one on the right)
2. With your arms extended and straight, place the palms of each hand respectively on the left and right chair
3. Support your full weight by lifting your legs and feet off the floor so your legs are straight and parallel to the floor

Execution

1. Shift your body weight (without moving your hands) so it is over your right arm
2. Lower yourself towards the floor (while inhaling) with most of your weight over your right arm until your right elbow bends 90 degrees
3. Legs remain straight and parallel to the floor
4. Torso can be straight up and down with elbows close to your body
5. As you push away from the floor, use your right arm for the majority of the pushing, using your left only for assistance, extend your arms, exhale, return to the top starting position
6. Shift your body weight so it is over your left arm and repeat the motion over your left side (when you have done a repetition once on the right and once on the left, this is considered just ONE complete repetition)
7. Repeat for a desired amount of repetitions per set

Body Parts Involved

Greater emphasis is placed on the side you happen to be leaning on.

1. Back of the upper arms (triceps)
2. Back of the shoulders (posterior deltoids)
3. Stomach area (abdominals)
4. If your body is straight up and down, some chest (pectorals) and some upper back (trapezius)
5. If your body is leaning forward, then more chest (pectorals)
6. If your body is leaning back, then more upper back (trapezius)

Side-to-Side, Top Starting, 2 – Point Dips
(Supported by both hands; feet and legs are suspended)

1

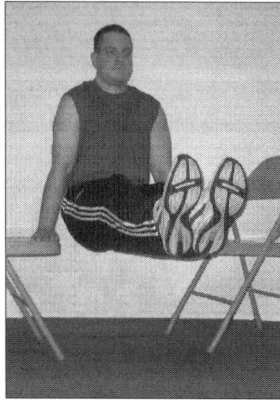

2

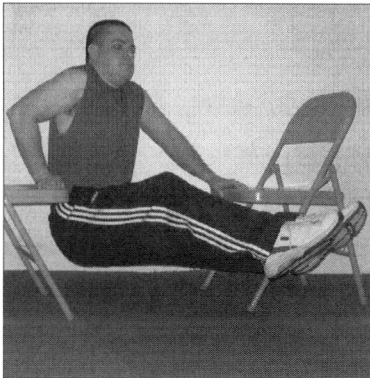

3

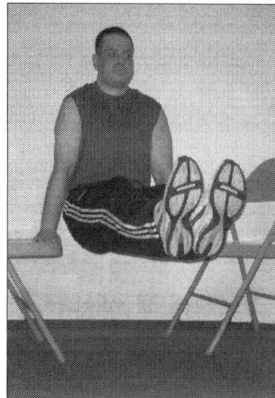

4

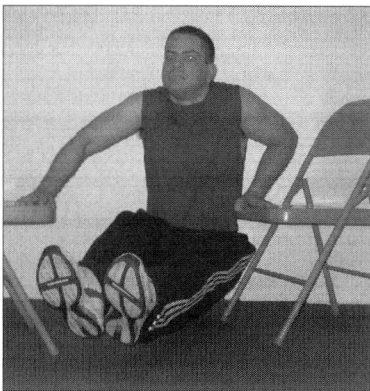

5

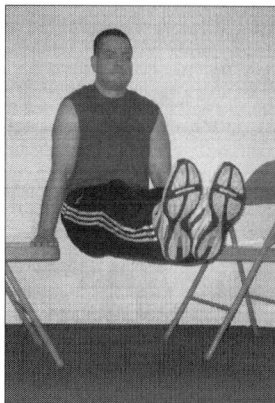

Side-to-Side, Bottom Starting, 2 – Point Dips
(Supported by both hands; feet and legs are suspended)

Starting Position

1. Place two chairs next to you (one on the left and one on the right)
2. With your arms bent 90 degrees, place the palms of each hand respectively on the left and right chair
3. Support your full weight by lifting your legs and feet off the floor so your legs are straight and parallel to the floor

Execution

1. Shift your body weight (without moving your hands) so it is by your right arm
2. As you push away from the floor, use your right arm for the majority of the pushing, using your left only for assistance, extend your arms and exhale
3. Now lower yourself towards the floor (while inhaling) with most of your weight over your right arm until your right elbow bends 90 degrees
4. Legs remain straight and parallel to the floor
5. Shift your body weight so it is by your left arm and repeat the motion over your left side (when you have done a repetition once on the right and once on the left, this is considered just ONE complete repetition)
6. Repeat for a desired amount of repetitions per set

Body Parts Involved

Greater emphasis is placed on the side you happen to be leaning on.

1. Back of the upper arms (triceps)
2. Back of the shoulders (posterior deltoids)
3. Stomach area (abdominals)
4. If your body is straight up and down, some chest (pectorals) and some upper back (trapezius)
5. If your body is leaning forward, then more chest (pectorals)
6. If your body is leaning back, then more upper back (trapezius)

Side-to-Side, Bottom Starting, 2 – Point Dips
(Supported by both hands; feet and legs are suspended)

1

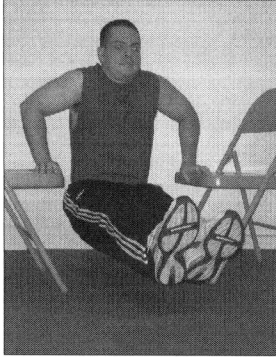

2

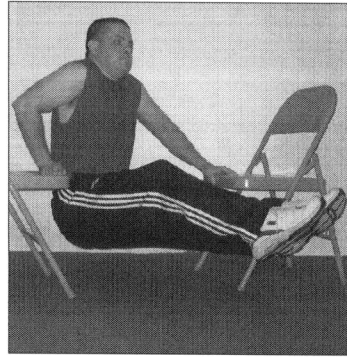

3

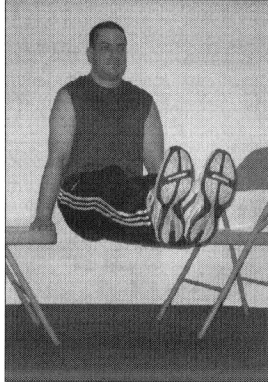

4

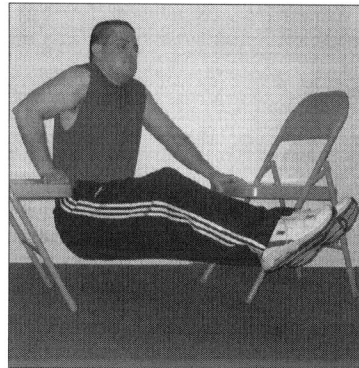

5

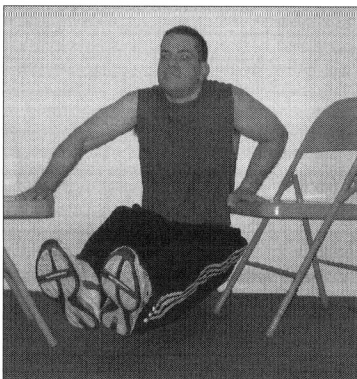

6

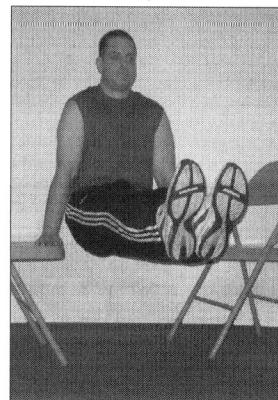

Pulling & Chinning

Standard 2 – Arm Pull Ups/Chin Ups

Starting Position

1. Grab an over head horizontal bar in either the overhand position (palms facing away; pull up position) or the underhand position (palms facing you; chin up position)
2. Hands should be about shoulder width apart
3. Arms should be straight and extended while you hang from the bar

Execution

1. Begin to pull yourself up towards the bar, while exhaling
2. For pull ups, elbows can be out towards the sides or in close to your body
3. For chin ups, elbows can be close to your body
4. At the top, your chin should be over the bar and the top of your chest should almost touch the bar
5. Lower yourself while inhaling and return to the starting position
6. Repeat for a desired amount of repetitions per set

Body Parts Involved

1. Sides of your back (latissimus dorsi)
2. Middle back (rhomboids)
3. Front of your upper arms (biceps)

Variations

1. **Hammer – Grip (Baseball Bat Grip) Pull Ups**
   a. Performed by gripping the bar just as gripping a baseball bat
   b. The bar will run above you from front-to-back instead of left-to-right
   c. As you reach the top, the head may be moved out of the way to either side

Note: Performing **chin ups** with hands in an underhand or supinated position (palms facing you) will result in greater emphasis of the biceps, as will bringing your hands closer together on the bar, with elbows tight by your sides. Performing **pull ups** with hands in an overhand or pronated position (palms facing away) will result in greater emphasis of the latissimus dorsi, as will placing your hands more than shoulder width apart and pointing your elbows out to the sides away from your body.

Standard 2 – Arm Pull Ups/Chin Ups

1
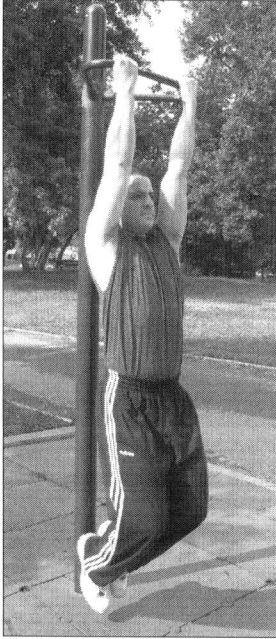

2
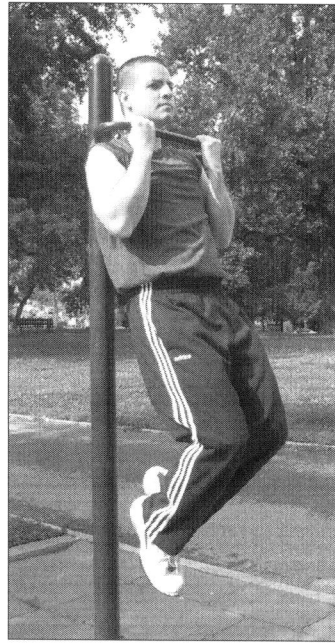

1
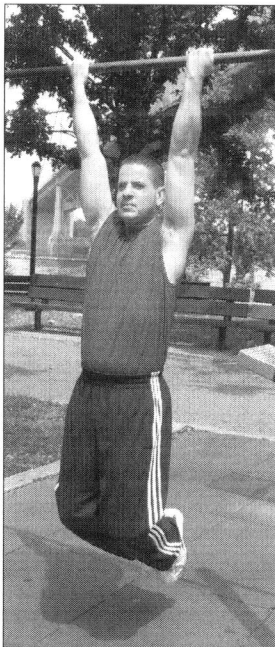

2
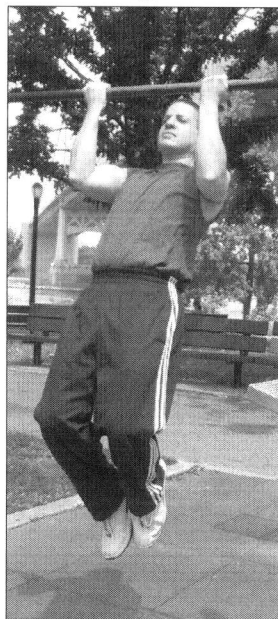

3
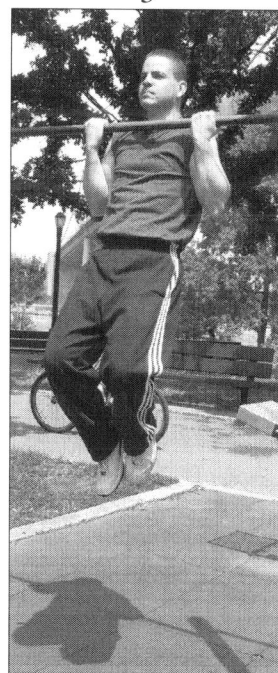

Side-to-Side, Bottom Starting, 2 – Arm Pull Ups/Chin Ups

Starting Position

1. Grab an over head horizontal bar in either the overhand position (palms facing away; pull up position) or the underhand position (palms facing you; chin up position)
2. Hands should be about shoulder width apart
3. Arms should be straight and extended while you hang from the bar

Execution

1. Shift your body weight so it is under your right arm
2. As you pull up towards the bar, use your right arm for the majority of the pulling, using your left arm only for assistance, bend your arms and exhale
3. At the top, your chin should be over the bar and the top of your chest should almost touch the bar
4. Now lower yourself towards the floor (while inhaling) with most of your weight under your right arm until your arms are straight and extended
5. Shift your body weight so it is under your left arm and repeat the motion under your left arm (when you have done a repetition once on the right and once on the left, this is considered just ONE complete repetition)
6. Repeat for a desired amount of repetitions per set

Body Parts Involved

Greater emphasis is placed on the side you are working on.

1. Sides of your back (latissimus dorsi)
2. Middle back (rhomboids)
3. Front of your upper arms (biceps)

Side-to-Side, Bottom Starting, 2 – Arm Pull Ups/Chin Ups

1

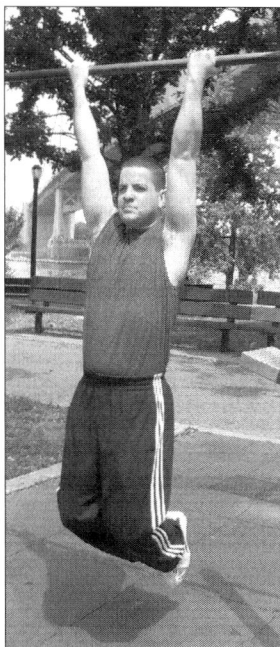

2

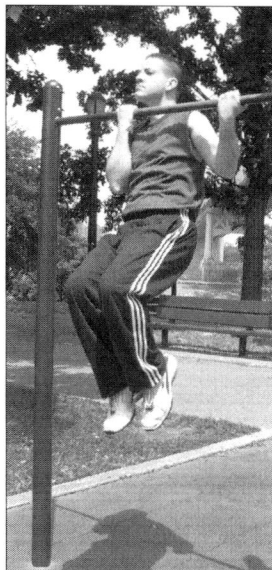

3

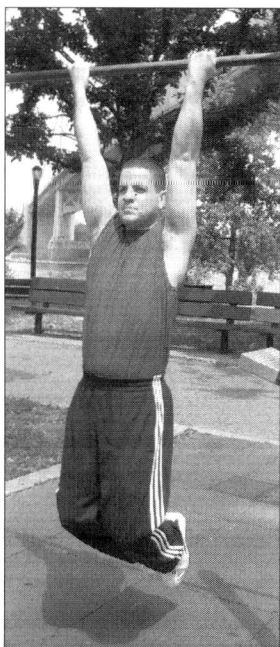

4

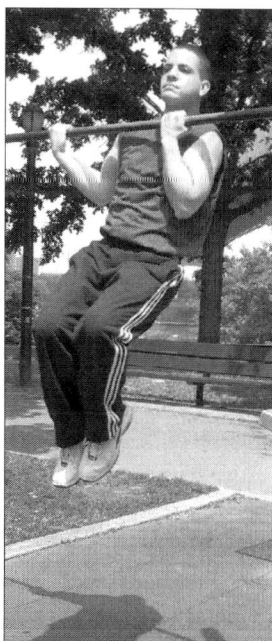

Side-to-Side, Top Starting, 2 – Arm Pull Ups/Chin Ups

Starting Position

1. Grab an over head horizontal bar in either the overhand position (palms facing away; pull up position) or the underhand position (palms facing you; chin up position)
2. Hands should be about shoulder width apart
3. Pull yourself up until your chin is over the bar and your chest is almost touching the bar

Execution

1. Shift your body weight so it is by your right arm
2. Lower yourself towards the floor (while inhaling) with most of your weight under your right arm until your arms are straight and extended
3. Now, as you pull up towards the bar, use your right arm for the majority of the pulling, using your left arm only for assistance, bend your arms and exhale
4. At the top, your chin should be over the bar and the top of your chest should almost touch the bar
5. Shift your body weight so it is by your left arm and repeat the motion under your left arm (when you have done a repetition once on the right and once on the left, this is considered just ONE complete repetition)
6. Repeat for a desired amount of repetitions per set

Body Parts Involved

Greater emphasis is placed on the side you are working on.

1. Sides of your back (latissimus dorsi)
2. Middle back (rhomboids)
3. Front of your upper arms (biceps)

Side-to-Side, Top Starting, 2 – Arm Pull Ups/Chin Ups

1

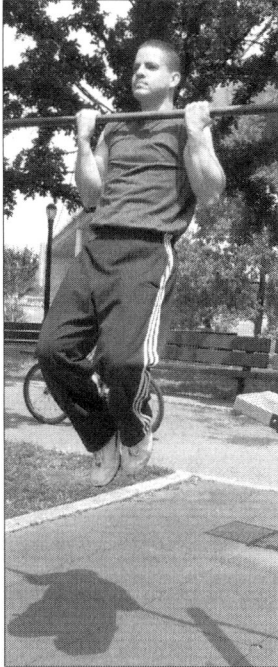

2

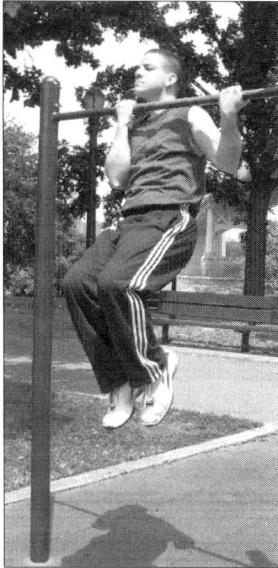

3

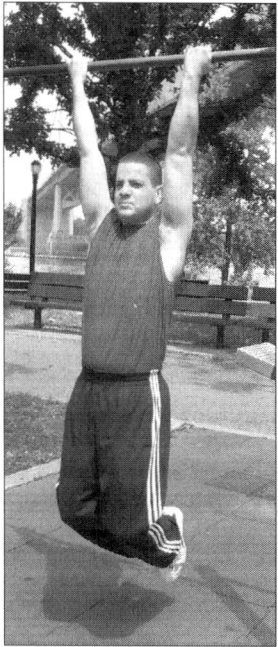

4

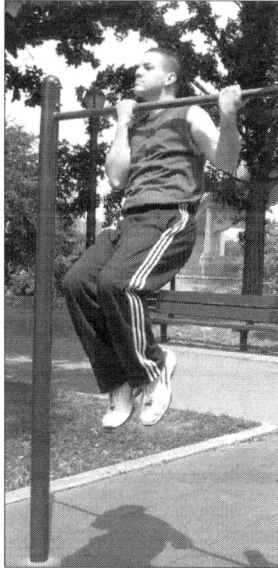

5

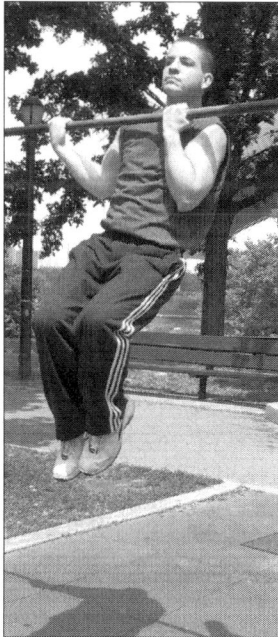

6

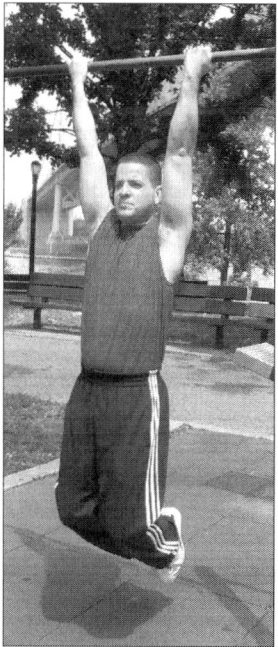

Assisted, 1 – Arm Pull Ups/Chin Ups

Starting Position

1. Grab an over head horizontal bar in either the overhand position (palms facing away; pull up position) or the underhand position (palms facing you; chin up position) with your right hand
2. Using your left arm as the assisting arm, grab the bar (overhand or underhand) with anywhere from 1 to 4 fingers
3. Hands should be about shoulder width apart
4. Arms should be straight and extended while you hang from the bar

Execution

1. Shift your body weight so it is under your right arm
2. As you pull up towards the bar, use your right arm for the majority of the pulling, using your left arm only for assistance, bend your arms and exhale
3. At the top, your chin should be over the bar and the top of your chest should almost touch the bar
4. Now lower yourself towards the floor (while inhaling) with most of your weight under your right arm until your arms are straight and extended
5. Repeat for a desired amount of repetitions per set
6. Switch to your left side, using your right hand for assistance with 1 to 4 fingers and repeat

Body Parts Involved

Greater emphasis is placed on the side you are working on.

1. Sides of your back (latissimus dorsi)
2. Middle back (rhomboids)
3. Front of your upper arms (biceps)

Note: When trying to progress to the **1 – arm, unassisted pull up/chin up**, it is best to start with four fingers on the assisting hand and slowly progress to using just one finger for assistance.

Assisted, 1 – Arm Pull Ups/Chin Ups

1

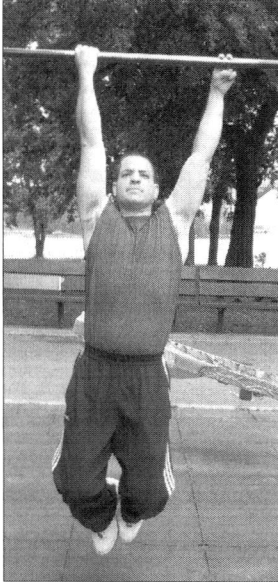

2

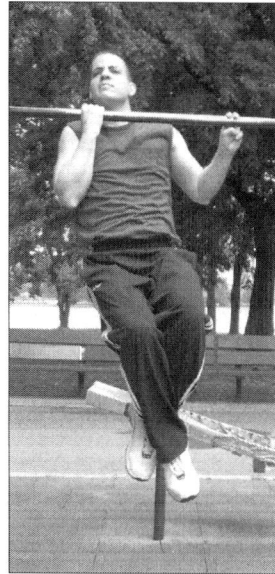

3

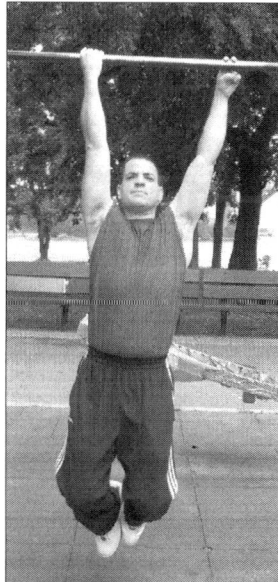

Assisted, 1 – Arm Pull Ups/Chin Ups
(with non-assisted negative)

Starting Position

1. Grab an over head horizontal bar in either the overhand position (palms facing away; pull up position) or the underhand position (palms facing you; chin up position) with your right hand
2. Using your left arm as the assisting arm, grab the bar (overhand or underhand) with anywhere from 1 to 4 fingers
3. Hands should be about shoulder width apart
4. Arms should be straight and extended while you hang from the bar

Execution

1. Shift your body weight so it is under your right arm
2. As you pull up towards the bar, use your right arm for the majority of the pulling, using your left arm only for assistance, bend your arms and exhale
3. At the top, your chin should be over the bar and the top of your chest should almost touch the bar
4. Release the grip on the bar from your left fingers so you are hanging completely from your right arm
5. Now lower yourself towards the floor (while inhaling) with all of your weight under your right arm until your arm is straight and extended
6. Repeat for a desired amount of repetitions per set
7. Switch to your left side, using your right hand for assistance with 1 to 4 fingers and repeat

Body Parts Involved

Greater emphasis is placed on the side you are working on.

1. Sides of your back (latissimus dorsi)
2. Middle back (rhomboids)
3. Front of your upper arms (biceps)

Assisted, 1 – Arm Pull Ups/Chin Ups
(with non-assisted negative)

1

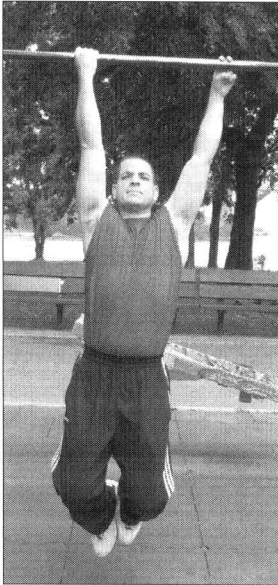

2

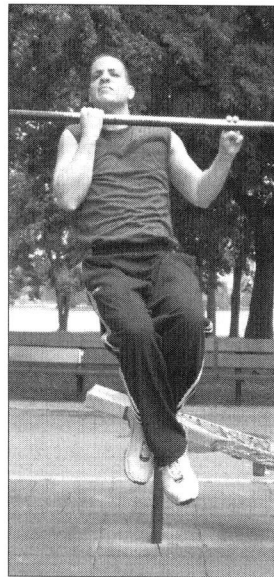

3

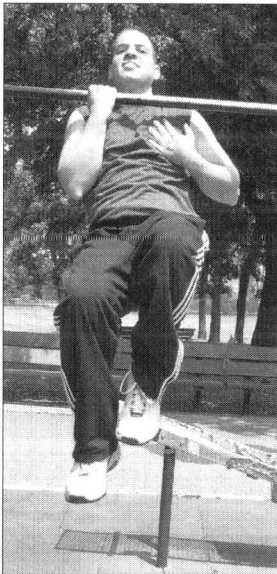

4

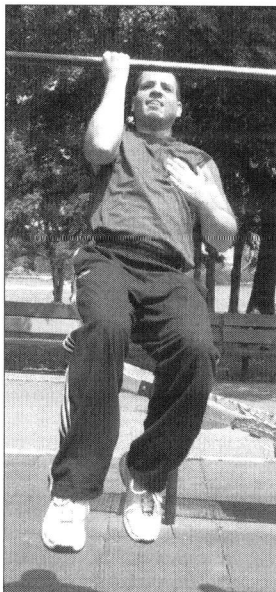

5

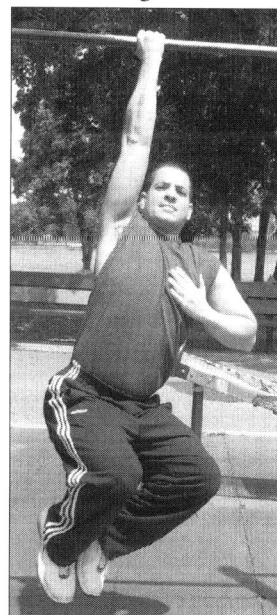

1 – Arm Pull Ups/Chin Ups

Starting Position

1. Grab an over head horizontal bar in either the overhand position (palms facing away; pull up position) or the underhand position (palms facing you; chin up position) with your right hand
2. Left hand may be placed anywhere, for balance, or just slightly touching the bar to prevent yourself from spinning
3. Right arm should be preferably straight and extended while you hang from the bar
4. Shoulder should be tight to your body and surrounding muscles tensed for support of the entire shoulder girdle (elbow may be slightly bent to facilitate the tension and support of the shoulder girdle)

Execution

1. Begin to pull yourself up towards the bar, while exhaling
2. Elbow will be close to your body
3. The entire muscles of your right arm, chest, abdominals, and back should be tensed
4. At the top, your chin should be over the bar and the top of your chest should almost touch the bar
5. Lower yourself while inhaling and return to the starting position
6. Repeat for a desired amount of repetitions per set
7. Switch to your left side and repeat

Body Parts Involved

All the emphasis is placed on the side you are working on.

1. Sides of your back (latissimus dorsi)
2. Middle back (rhomboids)
3. Front of your upper arms (biceps)

1 – Arm Pull Ups/Chin Ups

1

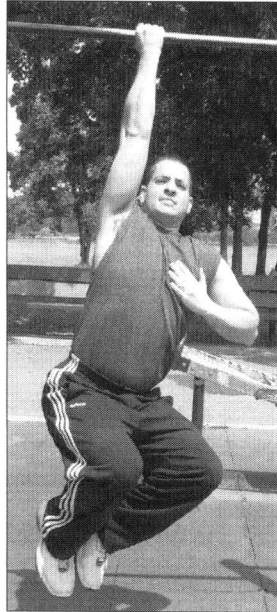

2

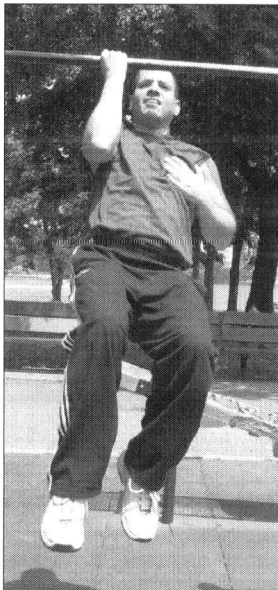

3

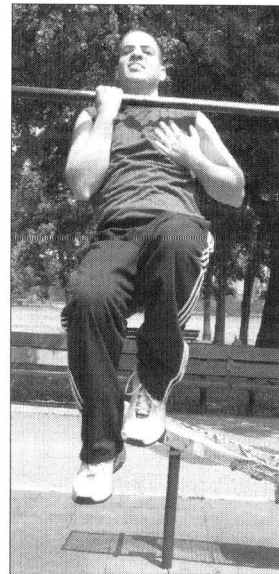

Horizontal Pull Ups (Knees over Chest)

Starting Position

1. Grab an over head horizontal bar in the overhand position (palms facing away; pull up position) and not the underhand position, as this will increase the amount of power you can generate during this exercise
2. Hands will be slightly wider than shoulder width apart
3. Arms should be straight and extended while you hang from the bar
4. Bring your knees to your chest and lift your hips to the level of your shoulders
5. Your back will be flat and horizontal with the floor; shoulders and hips will be on the same horizontal plane; knees will be over your chest and arms will be extended and straight
6. This starting position is known as the Tuck Front Lever

Execution

1. Begin to pull yourself up towards the bar, while exhaling
2. Elbows will be close to your body
3. Maintain a straight, horizontal back
4. At the top, your shins will touch the bar
5. Lower yourself while inhaling and return to the starting position
6. Repeat for a desired amount of repetitions per set

Body Parts Involved

1. Sides of your back (latissimus dorsi)
2. Middle back (rhomboids)
3. Front of your upper arms (biceps)
4. Back of your upper arms (triceps)
5. Stomach area (abdominals)
6. Back of the shoulders (posterior deltoids)

Variations

1. **Knees over Hips**
   a. Knees are bent and over the hips, forming a 90 degree angle between your stomach and thighs throughout the starting position and execution
   b. At the top of the pulling motion, your chest will almost touch the bar
   c. All else remains the same
2. **Legs Straight**
   a. Legs are straight, and entire body is horizontal during the starting position and execution
   b. At the top of the pulling motion, your chest will almost touch the bar
   c. All else remains the same

These variations increasingly stress the body parts involved.

Horizontal Pull Ups (Knees over Chest)

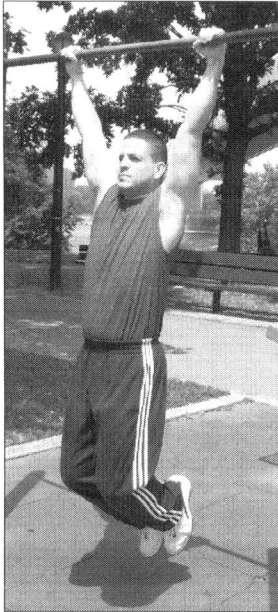

1

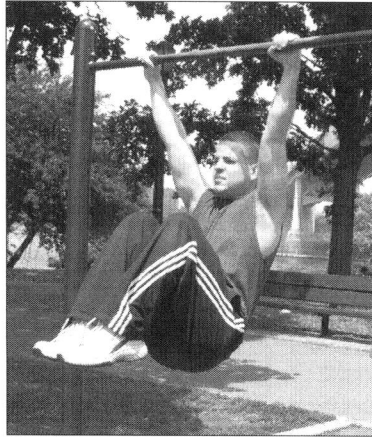

2

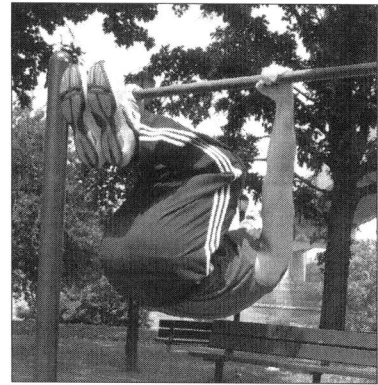

3

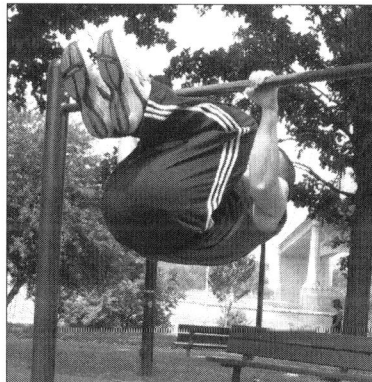

4

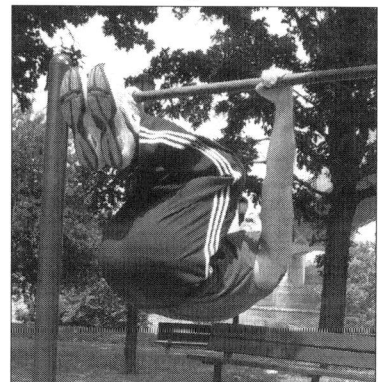

5

Leg Pressing
Prowess

Standard Squats

Starting Position

1. Stand with feet shoulder width apart and toes pointing straight forward or about 20 degrees to the sides

Execution

1. Face forward and keep your back straight as you begin to bend your knees and lower yourself towards the floor
2. Inhale as you lower yourself into a seated position
3. Try to keep your back vertical and straight, though leaning slightly forward is acceptable and natural
4. Your hands may be placed 1 to 2 feet in front of your chest for balance purposes throughout the movement
5. When you have reached a point where your thighs are parallel to the floor, begin to exhale as you raise yourself towards the starting position
6. Feet remain flat on the floor throughout the exercise
7. Repeat for a desired amount of repetitions per set

Body Parts Involved

1. Front of the thighs (quadriceps)
2. Back of the thighs (hamstrings)
3. Buttocks (gluteus maximus and medius)

Note: When you have reached a point when your thighs are parallel with the floor, your hips will be at the same height as your knees. For variety, it is safe and acceptable to drop your hips to a point below your knees if you wish to do so. Doing so will work the hamstrings and glutes harder than if you stop when your hips are level with your knees.

Standard Squats

1

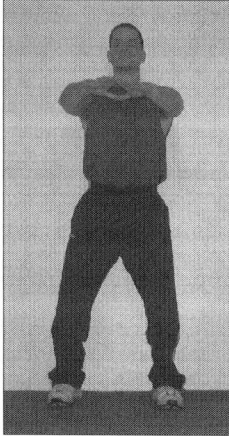

1a

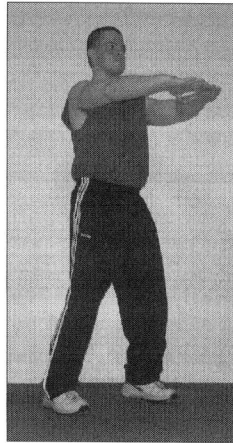

2

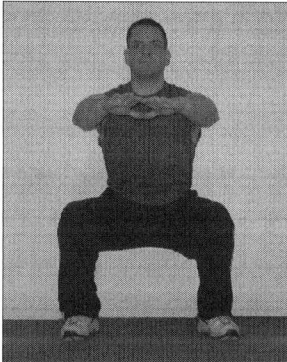

2a

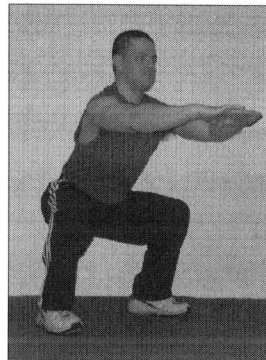

3

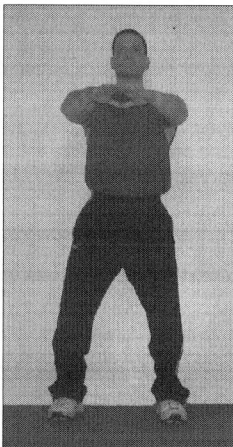

3a

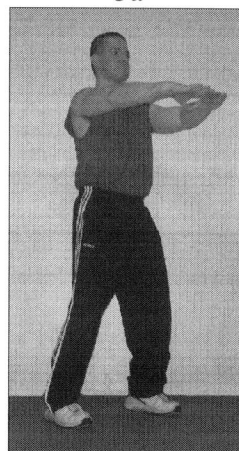

Wide Squats

Starting Position

1. Stand with feet 1 ½ to 2 shoulder widths apart and toes pointing out about 45 degrees to the sides

Execution

1. Face forward and keep your back straight as you begin to bend your knees and lower yourself towards the floor
2. Inhale as you lower yourself into a seated position with your knees pointing in the same direction as your toes
3. Your back should remain vertical throughout the movement and even form a slight arch in your lower back at the bottom of the movement
4. Your hands may be placed 1 to 2 feet in front of your chest for balance purposes throughout the movement
5. When you have reached a point where your thighs are parallel to the floor, begin to exhale as you raise yourself towards the starting position
6. Feet remain flat on the floor throughout the exercise
7. Repeat for a desired amount of repetitions per set

Body Parts Involved

1. Front of the thighs (quadriceps)
2. Back of the thighs (hamstrings)
3. Buttocks (gluteus maximus and medius)

Note: As in the standard squats, when you have reached a point when your thighs are parallel with the floor, your hips will be at the same height as your knees. For variety, it is safe and acceptable to drop your hips to a point below your knees if you wish to do so. Doing so will work the hamstrings and glutes harder than if you stop when your hips are level with your knees.

Wide Squats

1
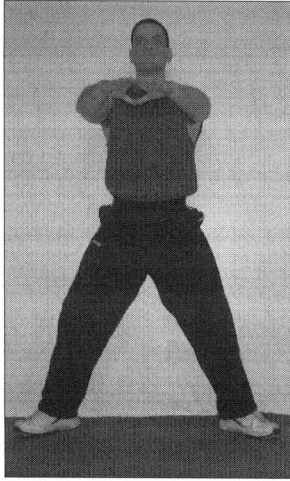

1a
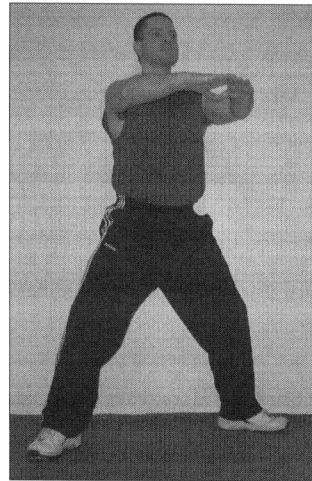

2
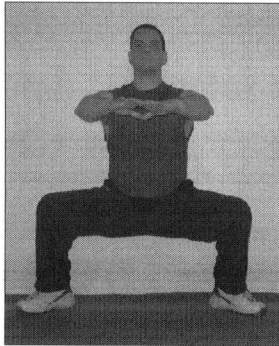

2a
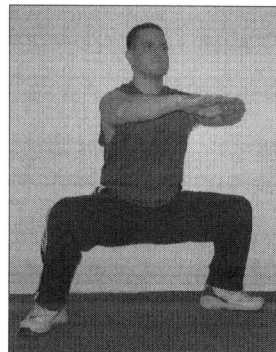

3
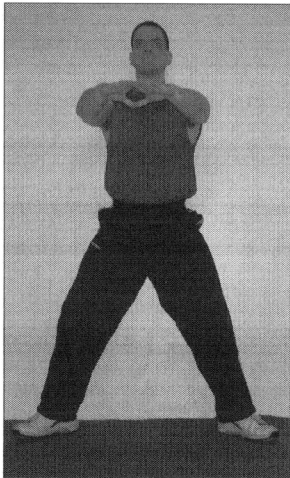

3a
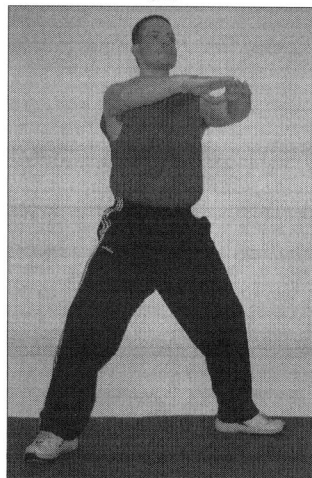

Forward Leg Lunges

Starting Position

1. Stand with feet shoulder width apart and toes pointing straight forward

Execution

1. Step forward with your right foot about 2 times your normal stride
2. As you inhale, begin to lower yourself towards the ground until both knees bend 90 degrees
3. At the bottom position, your back will be straight, though it is safe and normal if your shoulders are a little forward towards your front knee
4. Your front knee will be directly above your front toes, though (contrary to popular belief) it is safe if your knee extends a little forward of your front toes
5. As you exhale, push back off of your right foot and return to the starting position
6. Repeat all repetitions and sets on the right side
7. Switch to your left side and repeat

Body Parts Involved

1. Front of the thighs (quadriceps)
2. Back of the thighs (hamstrings)
3. Buttocks (gluteus maximus and medius)

Note: The greater the distance you cover on your step forward, the more you will emphasize the hamstrings and glutes.

Forward Leg Lunges

1

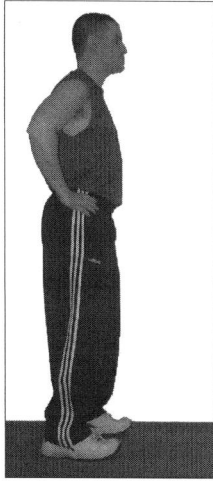

2

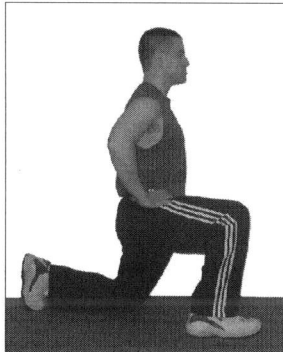

3

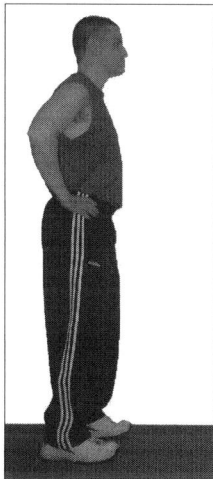

Chair Step Ups

Starting Position

1. Stand with feet shoulder width apart and toes pointing straight forward while facing a sturdy chair

Execution

1. Lift your right foot and place it on the center of the chair
2. Lean forward, only slightly, and exhale as you push yourself off the floor with your right leg
3. Your left leg will remain straight and behind your body during the movement
4. For balance purposes, you may initially grab onto the back of the chair as you begin your push upward
5. Once at the top, your right leg will be straight, and you can begin to inhale as you start bending your right leg and begin your decent towards the floor
6. When your left foot is flat on the ground you may repeat the exercise for a desired amount of repetitions per set
7. Switch to your left side and repeat

Body Parts Involved

1. Front of the thighs (quadriceps)
2. Back of the thighs (hamstrings)
3. Buttocks (gluteus maximus and medius)

Note: The higher the chair, or the higher your knee is from the level of your hips, the more you will emphasize the hamstrings and glutes.

Chair Step Ups

1

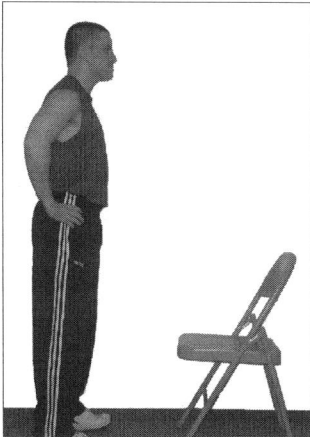

2

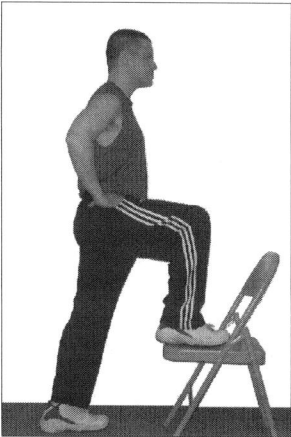

3

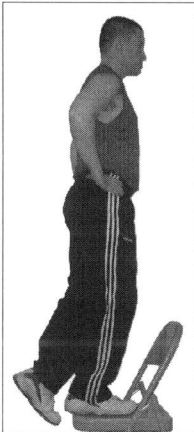

4

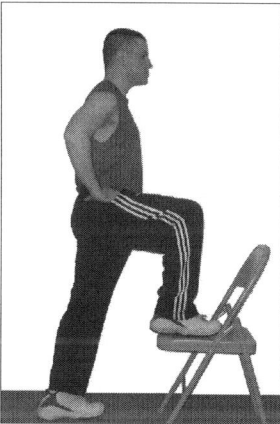

5

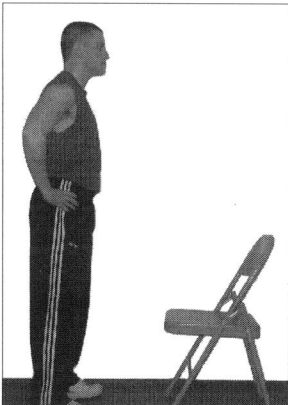

Single Leg Forward Squats

Starting Position

1. Stand with feet shoulder width apart and toes pointing straight forward
2. Bend your left knee 90 degrees or more so your left foot is behind you

Execution

1. While inhaling, bend your right leg until your thigh is near parallel with the floor
2. Your body will bend forward at the hips while your left foot raises behind you for balance
3. At the bottom, both hands should touch the floor
4. Exhale while you push against the floor with your right leg and return to the starting position
5. Repeat for a desired amount of repetitions per set
6. Switch to your left side and repeat

Body Parts Involved

1. Front of the thighs (quadriceps)
2. Back of the thighs (hamstrings)
3. Buttocks (gluteus maximus and medius)

Single Leg Forward Squats

1

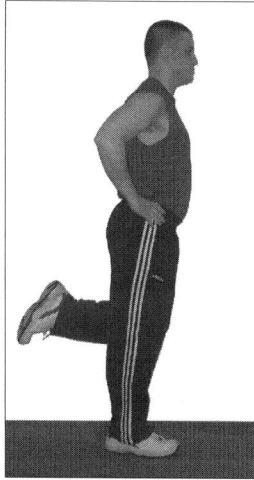

2

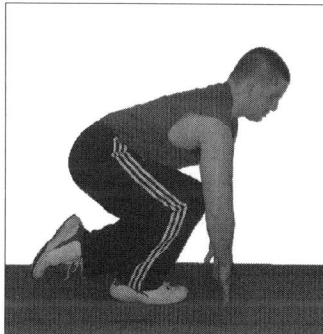

3

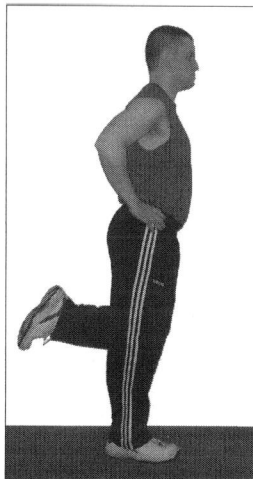

Assisted, 1 – Legged Squats
(with chair sitting)

Starting Position

1. With a chair behind you, stand with feet shoulder width apart and toes pointing straight forward
2. Place your left foot about 1 foot in front of you with toes touching the floor and heel off the floor

Execution

1. Placing most of your weight over your right leg (with right foot flat on the floor), bend your right knee as you lower your hips toward the chair
2. With your left heel off the floor, your left leg is only assisting and supports only a small amount of your weight
3. Inhale all the way down until you are seated in the chair
4. Exhale while you push against the floor with your right leg and return to the starting position
5. Repeat for a desired amount of repetitions per set
6. Switch to your left side and repeat

Body Parts Involved

1. Front of the thighs (quadriceps)
2. Back of the thighs (hamstrings)
3. Buttocks (gluteus maximus and medius)

Note: The lower the chair, meaning the lower you will have to travel downward, the more you will emphasize working the hamstrings and glutes.

Assisted, 1 – Legged Squats (with chair sitting)

1

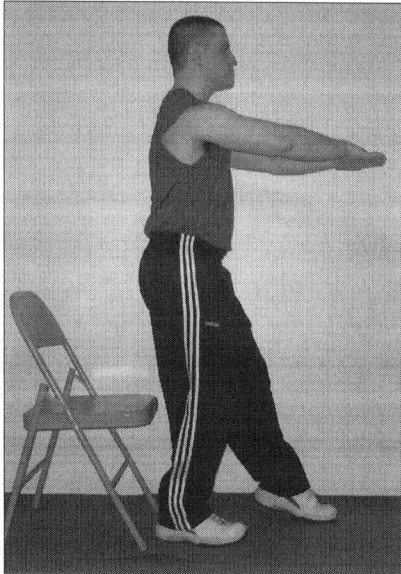

2

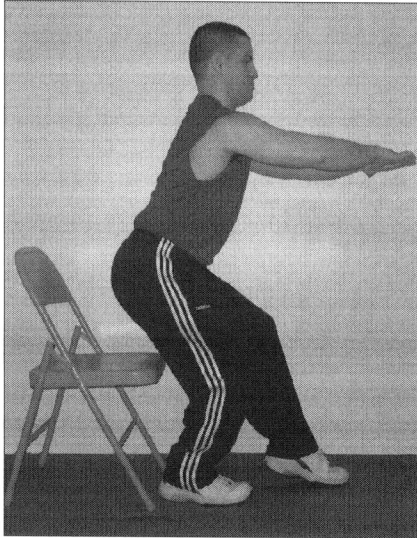

3

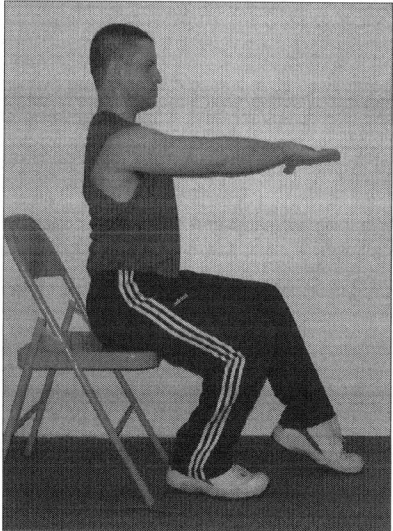

4

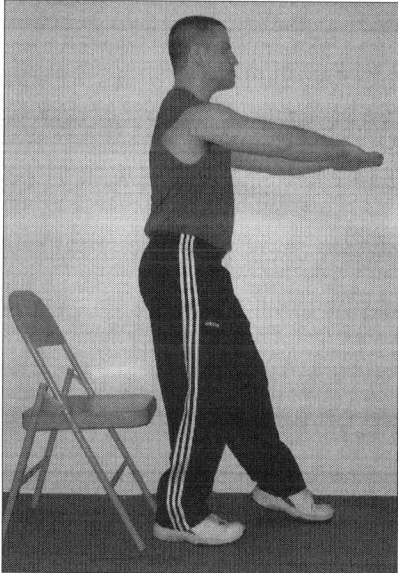

1 – Legged Squats (with chair sitting)

Starting Position

1. With a chair behind you, stand with feet shoulder width apart and toes pointing straight forward
2. Lift and extend your left knee so your entire left leg is straight, parallel with the ground, and at the level of your hip

Execution

1. Placing all of your weight over your right leg (with right foot flat on the floor), bend your right knee as you lower your hips toward the chair
2. Your left leg remains straight and parallel with the floor
3. Inhale all the way down until you are seated in the chair
4. Exhale while you push against the floor with your right leg and return to the starting position
5. Repeat for a desired amount of repetitions per set
6. Switch to your left side and repeat

Body Parts Involved

1. Front of the thighs (quadriceps)
2. Back of the thighs (hamstrings)
3. Buttocks (gluteus maximus and medius)

Note: The lower the chair, meaning the lower you will have to travel downward, the more you will emphasize working the hamstrings and glutes.

1 – Legged Squats (with chair sitting)

1

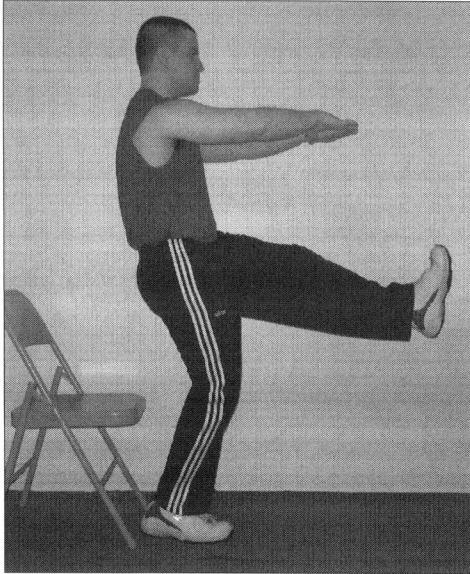

2

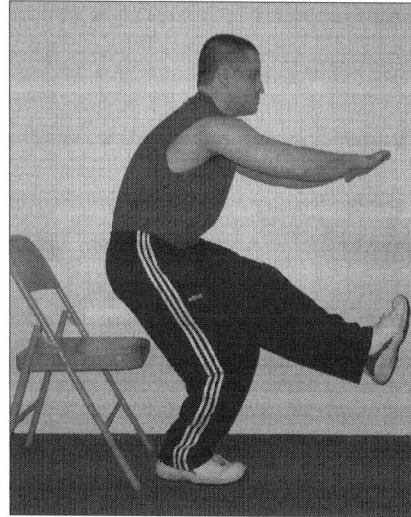

3

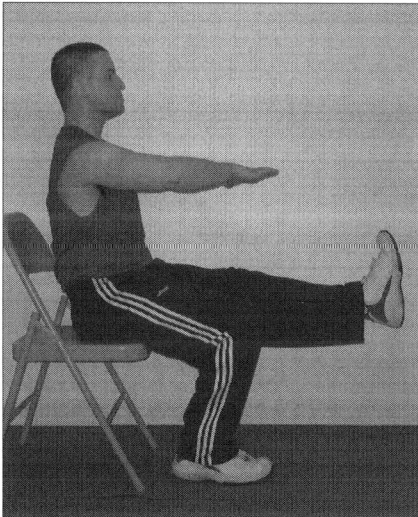

4

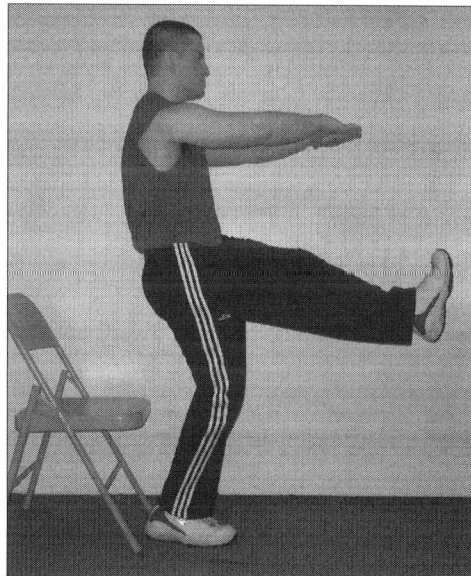

1 – Legged Squats (Pistols)

Starting Position

1. Stand with feet shoulder width apart and toes pointing straight forward
2. Lift and extend your left knee so your entire left leg is straight, parallel with the ground, and at the level of your hip

Execution

1. Placing all of your weight over your right leg (with right foot flat on the floor), bend your right knee as you lower your hips toward the floor
2. Your left leg remains straight and parallel with the floor
3. Inhale all the way down until your hips drop below the level of your knee
4. Exhale while you push against the floor with your right leg and return to the starting position
5. Repeat for a desired amount of repetitions per set
6. Switch to your left side and repeat

Body Parts Involved

1. Front of the thighs (quadriceps)
2. Back of the thighs (hamstrings)
3. Buttocks (gluteus maximus and medius)

1 – Legged Squats (Pistols)

1

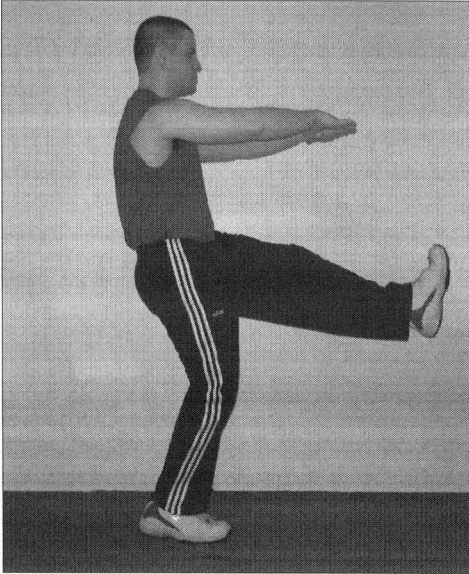

2

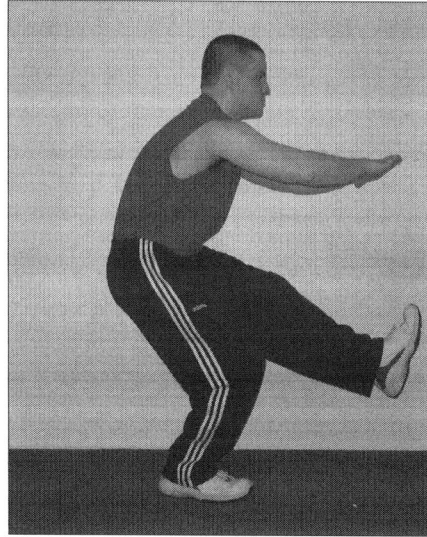

3

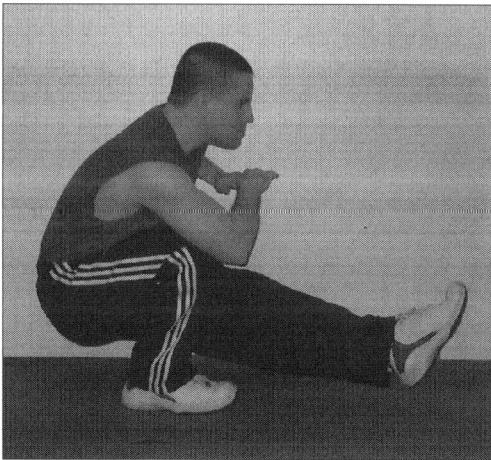

4

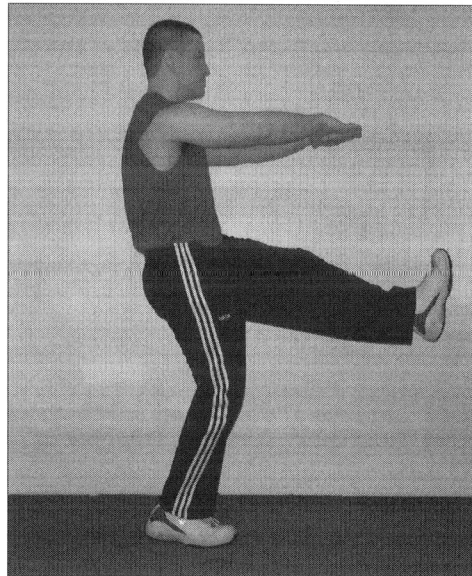

Leg Curling
Conditioning

2 – Legged Curls
(with arm assistance)

Starting Position

1. Position yourself flat on the ground with your chest to the floor
2. Make sure your feet are held in place by placing them comfortably under a heavy object that is slightly elevated off the ground (such as underneath a couch or stable dresser), or have a partner hold your feet down
3. Place both hands at about chest level, as if ready to perform a standard push up

Execution

1. Begin to bend your knees as if you want to lift the object or partner holding your feet down (for safety concerns, make sure the object holding your feet down is immovable with the force you are applying)
2. As you bend your knees more forcefully, your body (from your knees to your head) should start to raise off the floor with as little assistance from your arms as possible
3. Exhale as your body is rising, keeping perfectly straight between your knees and head
4. Use your arms as needed, making sure most of the effort is being applied by your legs
5. When you reach a position where your body is vertical, begin to lower yourself down while inhaling and using your arms for assistance until your chest reaches the floor
6. Repeat for a desired amount of repetitions per set

Body Parts Involved

1. Back of the thighs (hamstrings)
2. Lower Back (sacrospinalis)

Variations

1. **2 – Legged Curls (no arm assistance)**
   Same, but without any assistance from your arms
2. **1 – Legged Curls (with arm assistance)**
   Same, but one leg is held in place, while the other leg is bent 90 degrees and is freely movable
3. **1 – Legged Curls (no arm assistance)**
   Same, but one leg is held in place, while the other leg is bent 90 degrees and is freely movable with no assistance from your arms

2 – Legged Curls (with arm assistance)

1

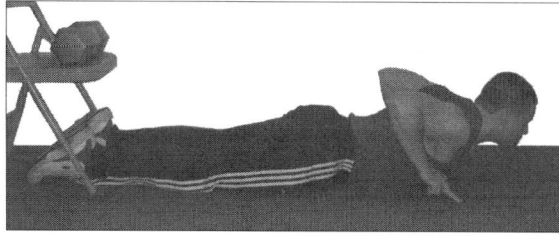

2

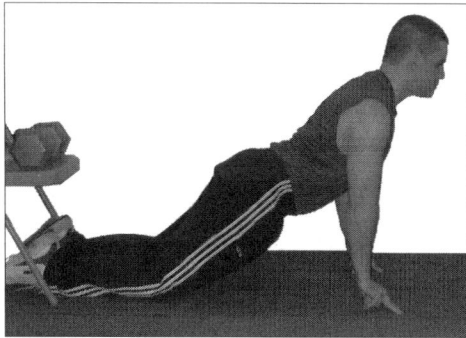

3

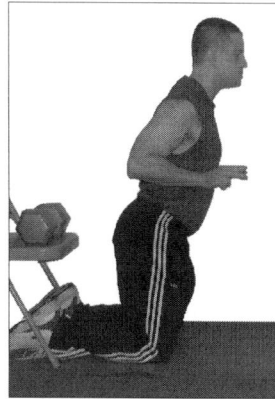

2 – Legged Curls (no arm assistance)

1

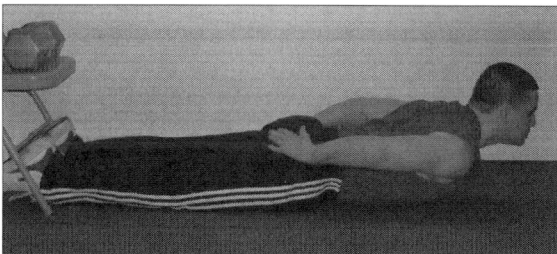

2

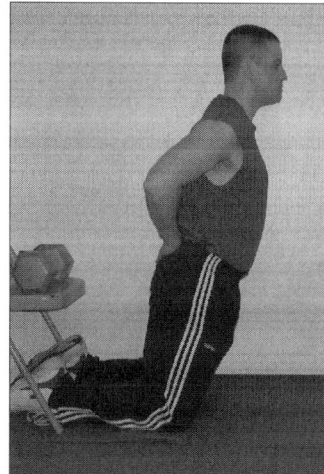

Reverse Leg Curls

Starting Position

1. Kneel down on the floor with your feet together, and knees slightly apart
2. The lower half of your legs from toes to knees are flat on the ground
3. The rest of your body from knees to head is in a vertical position
4. Arms can rest by your sides

Execution

1. As you inhale, begin to lean your body back and bend at the knees, keeping your torso tight and back straight
2. When you have reached your maximum bottom position, exhale as you begin to raise your body and lean forward
3. Return to the starting position
4. Repeat for a desired amount of repetitions per set

Body Parts Involved

1. Front of the thighs (quadriceps)
2. Front of the hips (hip flexors)
3. Stomach area (abdominals)

Note: If you cannot lean back as much as you would like, use an arm for assistance by slightly turning to the right when you reach your maximum bottom position and use your right arm to assist you in lowering yourself a little more. Use the same arm to assist in pushing yourself back up. Now immediately repeat on the left side. Not only will you maximize your bottom position, but the twisting from side to side will work the oblique muscles of your abdominals.

Reverse Leg Curls

1

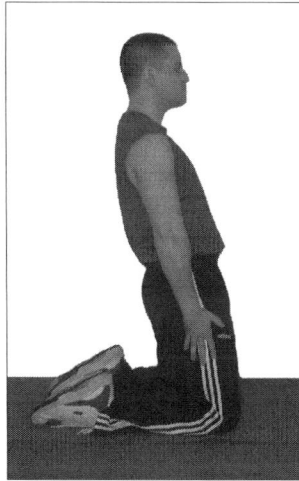

2

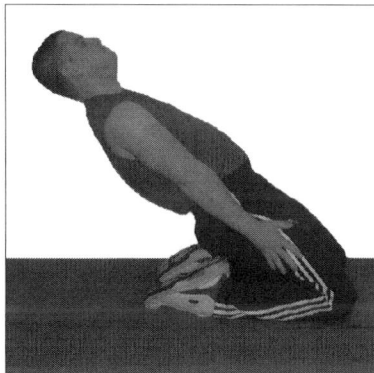

Reverse Leg Curls (with arm assistance)

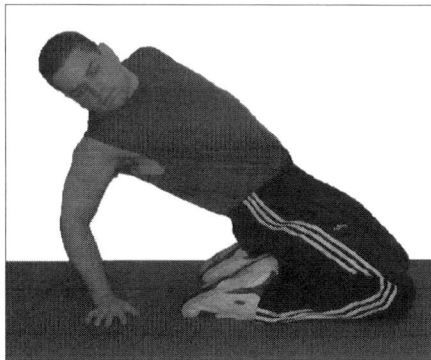

Calf Development

2 – Legged Calf Raises

Starting Position

1. Standing with feet shoulder width apart, face the back of a chair
2. Place one hand on the back of the chair for balance only

Execution

1. Using both feet, exhale as you raise both heels of the floor to maximum height
2. Grab on to the back of the chair with one hand for balance purposes only
3. Inhale as you lower yourself down with both feet, to the starting position
4. Repeat for a desired amount of repetitions per set

Body Parts Involved

1. Calf muscle (gastrocnemius)

Variations

1. **1 – Legged Calf Raises**
   Perform as above using only one leg

Note: To increase the difficulty of the exercise, the 1 or 2 – legged calf raises can be performed by standing on a step, letting the heels hang over the edge of the step. The heels should drop below the level of your toes, thereby increasing the range of motion and distance your heel must travel to the top position. You should feel a gentle stretch of the calves as you stand in the starting position with heels dropping below the level of your toes. This increased range of motion adds difficulty to the exercise and works the calves more thoroughly.

2 – Legged Calf Raises

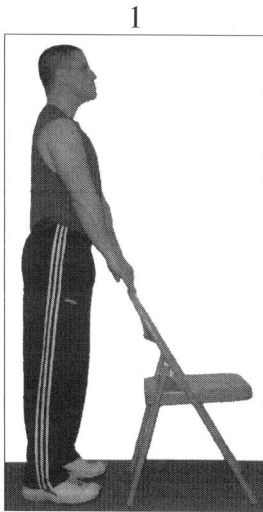

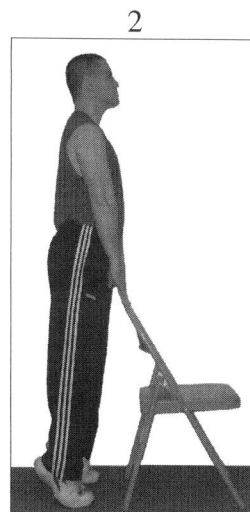

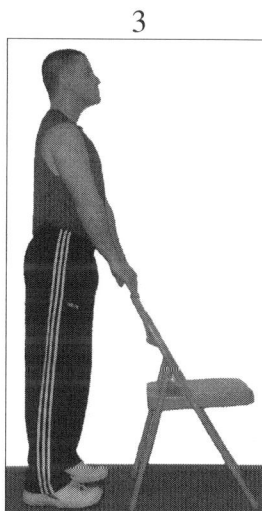

1

2

3

2 – Legged Calf Raises
(knees bent 90 degrees)

Starting Position

1. Stand with feet shoulder width apart and toes pointing forward
2. Bend your knees 90 degrees into a seated squat position

Execution

1. Using both feet, exhale as you raise both heels of the floor to maximum height
2. Both hands may be placed 1 to 2 feet away from your chest for balance purposes
3. Inhale as you lower yourself down with both feet to the starting position
4. Try to keep your knees at 90 degrees, meaning your hips should be moving up and down with the movement of your heels
5. Repeat for a desired amount of repetitions per set

Body Parts Involved

1. Front of the thighs (quadriceps)
2. Calf muscle (gastrocnemius)
3. Other calf muscle used more when knees are bent 90 degrees (soleus)

Variations

1. **1 – Legged Calf Raises (knees bent 90 degrees)**
   Same as above, except that one foot keeps the heel off the floor (using the toes for balance and assistance only) while the other foot is actively performing the exercise of raising and lowering the heel. Remember to switch sides.

2 – Legged Calf Raises
(knees bent 90 degrees)

1
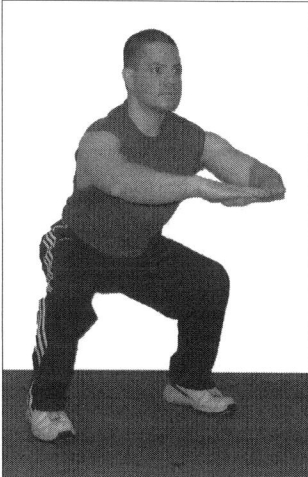

2
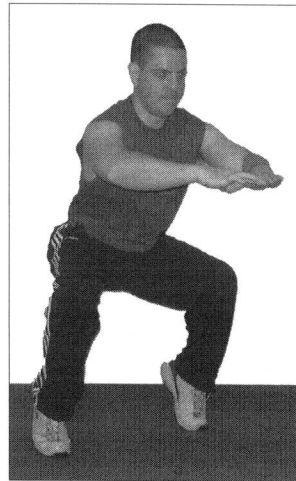

1 – Legged Calf Raises (knees bent 90 degrees)

1
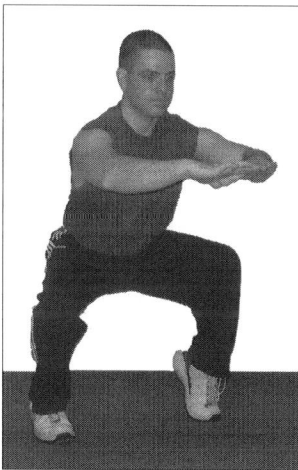

2
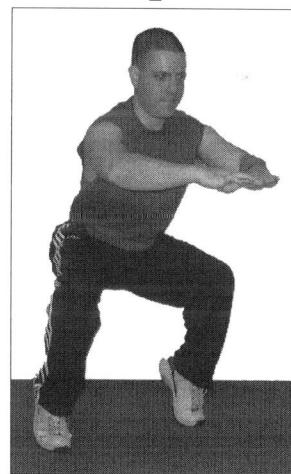

Tight Abs and a Strong Back

Crunches

Starting Position

1. Lie flat with your back on the floor
2. Knees are bent and feet remain flat on the floor
3. Arms are bent so the tips of your fingers are touching your ears

Execution

1. While exhaling, raise your chest until your shoulder blades are off the floor
2. At the same time, contract your abdominals as if trying to touch your elbows to your hips
3. Fingers remain touching your ears
4. Lower back remains flat on the floor
5. While inhaling, lower your shoulder blades back to the floor and return to the starting position
6. Repeat for a desired amount of repetitions per set

Body Parts Involved

1. Stomach area (abdominals)

1

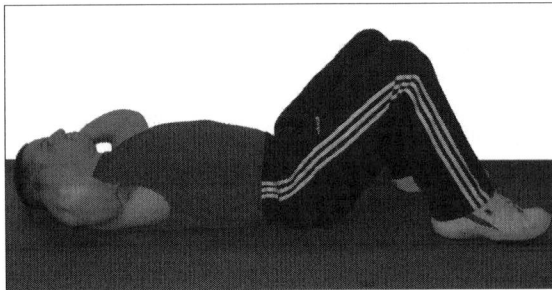

2

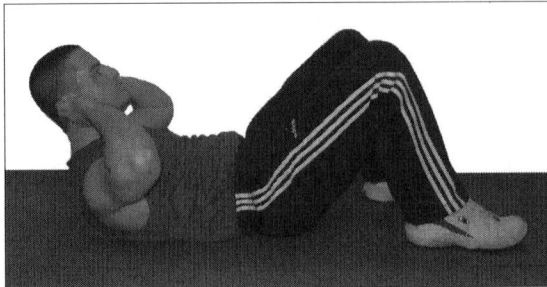

Oblique Crunches (Twisting)

Starting Position

1. Lie flat with your back on the floor
2. Knees are bent and feet remain flat on the floor
3. Arms are bent so the tips of your fingers are touching your ears

Execution

1. While exhaling, raise your chest until your shoulder blades are off the floor
2. At the same time, twist your torso to the right and contract your abdominals, trying to touch your left elbow to your right hip
3. Fingers remain touching your ears
4. Lower back remains flat on the floor
5. As you return to the starting position, inhale, and lower your shoulder blades back to the floor
6. Repeat for a desired amount of repetitions per set on one side
7. Switch to the other side and repeat

Body Parts Involved

1. Stomach area (abdominals)
2. Sides of your stomach (obliques)

1

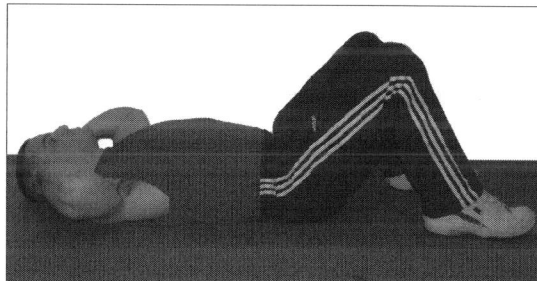

2

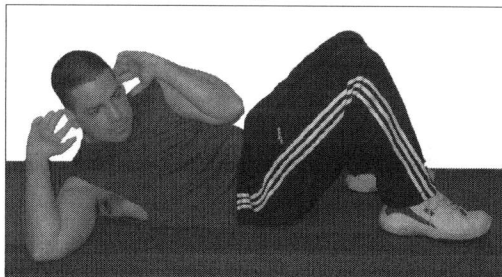

Oblique Crunches (Flat)

Starting Position

1. Lie flat with your back on the floor
2. Knees are bent and feet remain flat on the floor
3. Arms are bent so the tips of your fingers are touching your ears
4. Now twist your hips to the right so the right hip and entire right side of your right leg are flat on the floor
5. Left leg is resting flat on the right leg and knees are slightly bent
6. Try to keep both shoulder blades flat on the floor with chest pointing up

Execution

1. While exhaling, raise your chest until your shoulder blades are off the floor
2. At the same time, contract your abdominals and left side obliques as if trying to touch your elbows to your hips
3. Fingers remain touching your ears
4. Lower back remains flat on the floor
5. While inhaling, lower your shoulder blades back to the floor and return to the starting position
6. Repeat for a desired amount of repetitions per set
7. Switch sides so the left side of your left leg is flat on the floor and repeat to work your right side obliques

Body Parts Involved

1. Stomach area (abdominals)
2. Sides of your stomach (obliques)

1

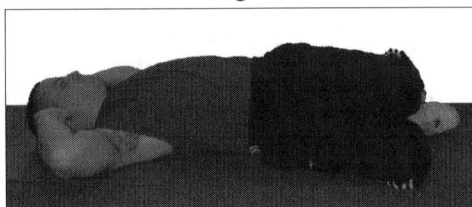

2

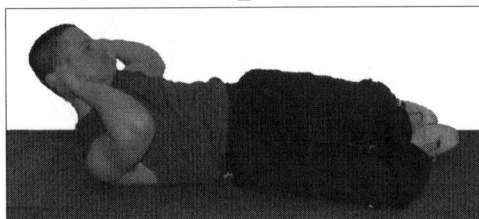

Reverse Crunches

Starting Position

1. Lie flat with your back on the floor
2. Legs are straight and bent at the hips so your legs are straight up-and-down while your torso is flat on the floor (your body should form an "L" shape)
3. Arms are by your side with hands by your hips, flat on the floor

Execution

1. Exhale while you elevate your hips off the floor and your feet attempt to reach towards the sky
2. Control your return to the starting position by contracting your lower abdominals
3. Inhale as you lower your hips
4. Repeat for a desired amount of repetitions per set

Body Parts Involved

1. Lower stomach area (lower abdominals)

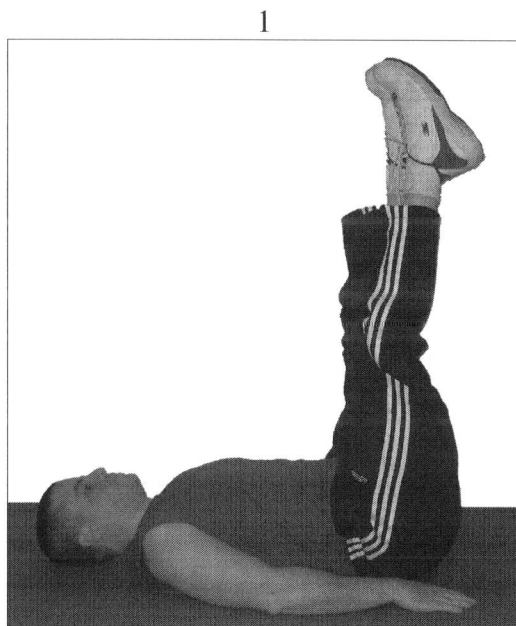

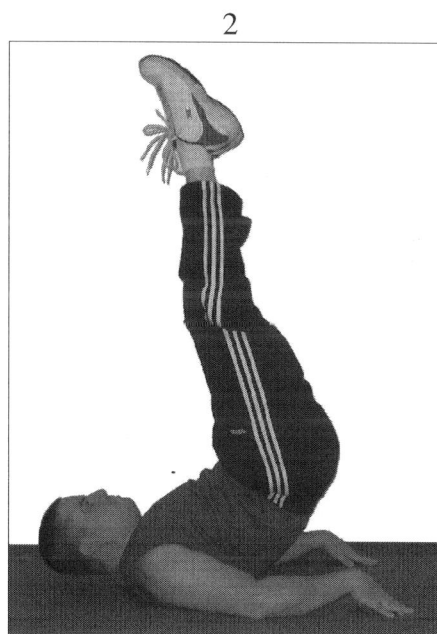

1

2

Janda Sit Ups

Starting Position

1. Lie flat with your back on the floor
2. Knees are bent and feet remain flat on the floor
3. Arms can be straight and elevated with the tips of your fingers attempting to reach over your knees

Execution

1. Completely tighten and tense the backs of your legs (hamstrings) and buttocks (glutes) – this is extremely important, as it serves to inactivate the hip flexors thereby assuring that only the abdominals are used during this sit up
2. While exhaling, flex your abdominals as you raise your entire torso off the floor and bring your chest to your knees
3. Keep the hamstrings and glutes tensed throughout the motion
4. Inhale on the way down as you return to the starting position
5. Repeat for a desired amount of repetitions per set

Body Parts Involved

1. Stomach area (abdominals)

1

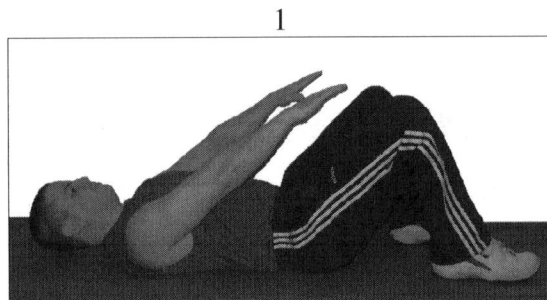

2

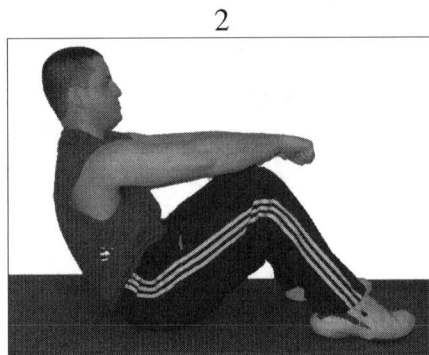

Pendulum Twists

Starting Position

1. Lie flat with your back on the floor
2. Legs are straight and bent at the hips so your legs are straight up-and-down while your torso is flat on the floor (your body should form an "L" shape)
3. Arms will be straight and away from your sides so they form a "T" shape with your torso

Execution

1. While keeping your legs straight, and exhaling, begin to twist your torso to the right until the right side of your right leg touches the floor
2. Inhale as your return to the starting position
3. Repeat on the left side
4. When you have twisted once to the right and once to the left, this is considered just one repetition
5. Repeat for a desired amount of repetitions per set

Body Parts Involved

1. Stomach area (abdominals)
2. Sides of your stomach (obliques)

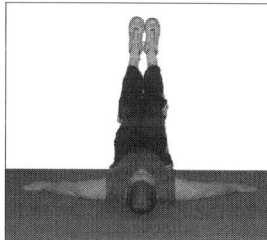

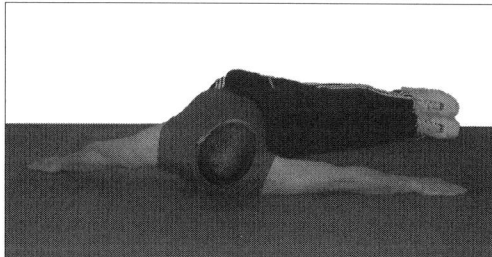
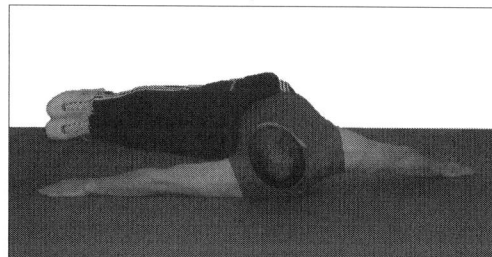

Lying Down Leg Lifts

Starting Position

1. Lie on your back, flat on the floor
2. Legs are straight and together
3. Arms are by your sides or place your hands under your buttocks for lower back support

Execution

1. While exhaling, keep your legs straight as you begin to raise them off the floor
2. Keep your lower back flat on the floor
3. Raise your legs until your hips form a 90 degree angle with the floor
4. Inhale as you lower your legs and return to the starting position
5. Repeat for a desired amount of repetitions per set

Body Parts Involved

1. Stomach area (abdominals)
2. Hips (hip flexors)
3. Front of your thighs (quadriceps)

1

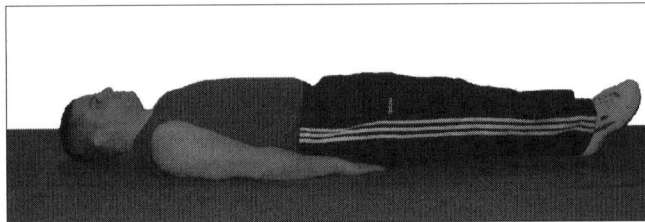

2

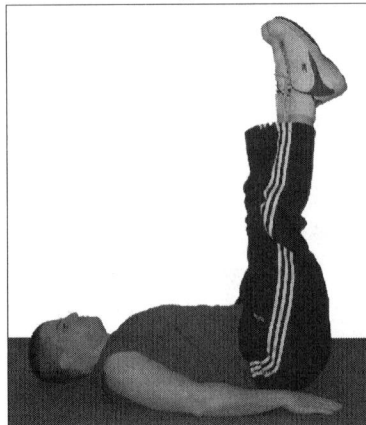

Hanging Knee Lifts

Starting Position

1. Hang from a bar with your body straight and legs straight down

Execution

1. Exhale as you begin to raise your knees
2. Raise your knees toward your chest by flexing your hips
3. Also, bend and flex your knees as you raise them so your heels come in front of your buttocks
4. Once your knees have reached their highest point, inhale as you lower them to the starting position
5. Repeat for a desired amount of repetitions per set

Body Parts Involved

1. Stomach area (abdominals)
2. Hips (hip flexors)

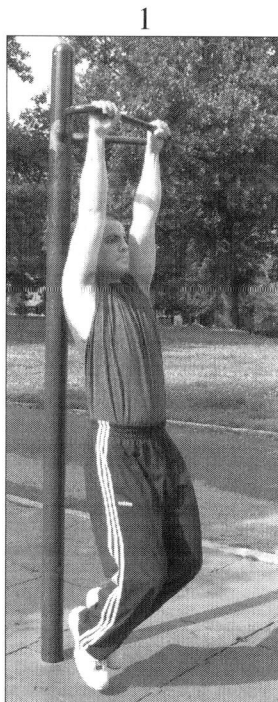

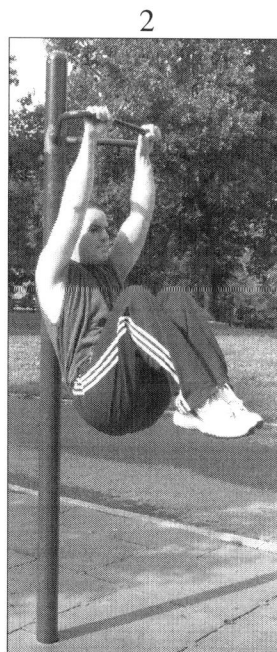

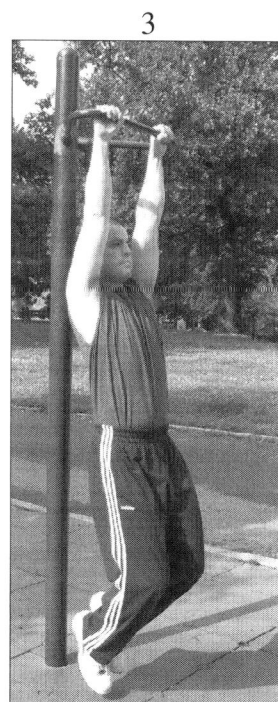

Hanging Leg Lifts

Starting Position

1. Hang from a bar with your body straight and your legs straight down

Execution

1. Keeping your legs straight, exhale as you flex your hips and slowly raise your legs
2. Continue to raise your straight legs, attempting to touch the bar with your feet
3. Once your feet have reached their highest position, inhale as you lower your straight legs to the starting position
4. Repeat for a desired amount of repetitions per set

Body Parts Involved

1. Stomach area (abdominals)
2. Hips (hip flexors)

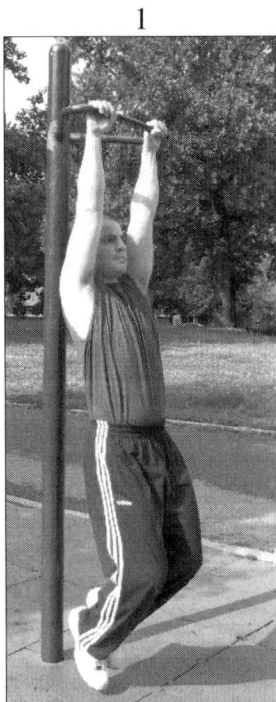

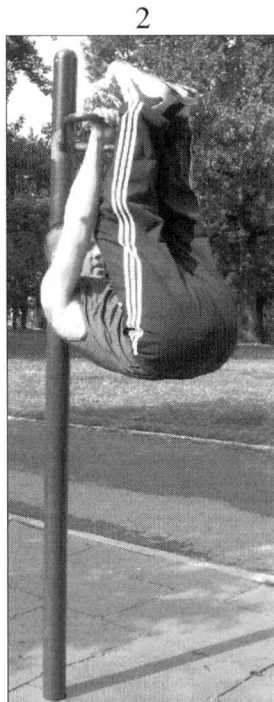

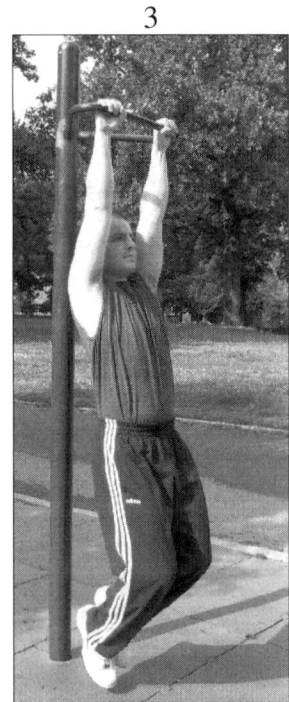

Supermans

Starting Position

1. Lie flat on your stomach with legs straight and arms in front of you (as if flying like Superman)

Execution

1. While exhaling, raise your arms, chest, and legs off the floor (keeping your arms and legs straight)
2. At the highest point, begin to inhale as you slowly lower your arms, chest and legs to the ground
3. Repeat for a desired amount of repetitions per set

Body Parts Involved

1. Lower back (sacrospinalis)

Variations

1. **Alternating Supermans**
   Same starting position except that you will lift the **right** arm, chest, and **left** leg for the desired repetitions per set, then switch to the alternate side and repeat

1

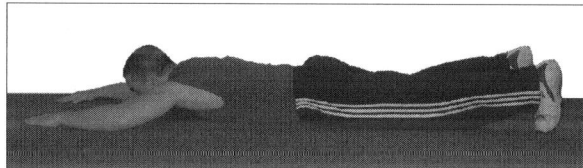

2

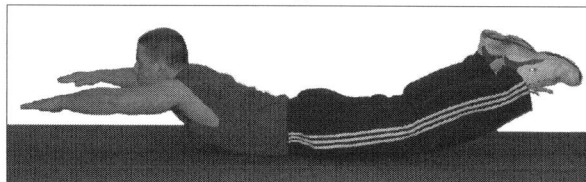

Alternating Supermans

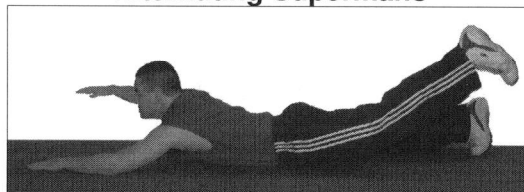

Back Extensions

Starting Position

1. Position a chair so the back of the chair is to your left or right side
2. Facing straight down, position yourself so the front of your thighs are flat on the seat of the chair, your upper body is hanging off the chair with your face looking down at the floor and your back being parallel to and facing the ceiling
3. Place the heels of your feet under an immovable piece of furniture, or have a partner hold your feet in place with toes pointing towards the floor
4. Bend at the hips and lower your upper body towards the floor
5. Place your hands so they are slightly touching your ears

Execution

1. With your torso low to the ground and bent at the hips, exhale as you raise your torso away from the ground
2. Extend your back upward, just past parallel with the floor
3. When you have reached your maximum height, inhale as you return to the starting position
4. Repeat for a desired amount of repetitions per set

Body Parts Involved

1. Lower back (sacrospinalis)
2. Back of your legs (hamstrings)

Variations

1. **Twisting Back Extensions**
   Same starting position except that you will twist your torso to the right side and maintain this turned position as you execute the extensions for the desired repetitions per set, then switch to the left side and repeat

Back Extensions

1

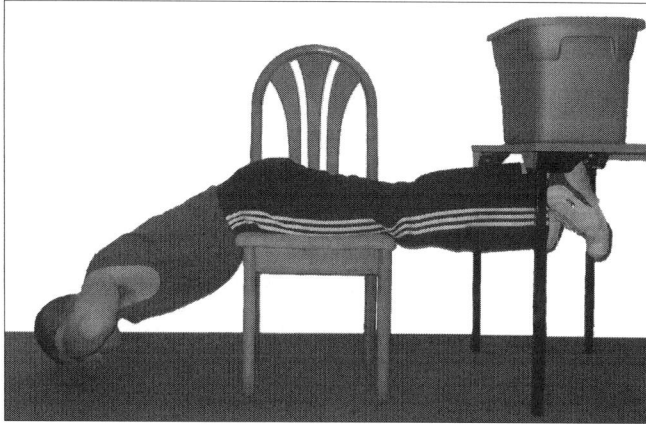

2

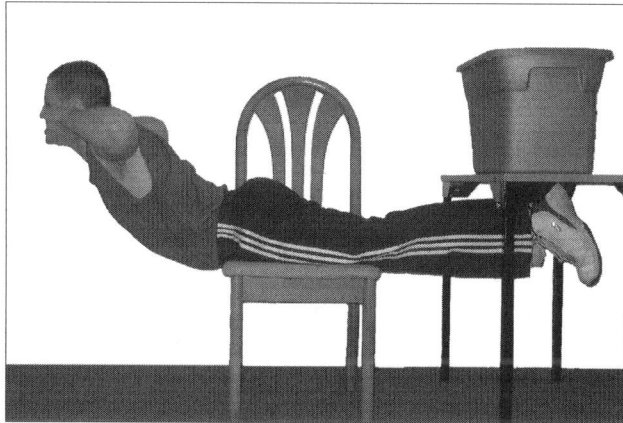

Twisting Back Extensions

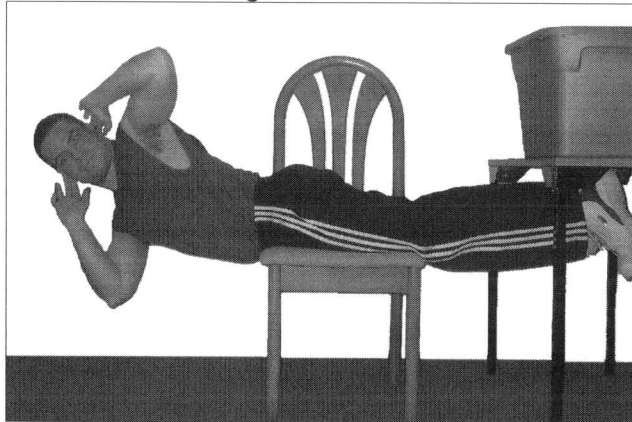

Ultimate Body Curling

Hanging Body Curls

Starting Position

1. Grab an over head horizontal bar in the overhand position (palms facing away)
2. Hands should be a little wider than shoulder width apart
3. Arms should be straight and extended while you hang from the bar

Execution

1. While exhaling, bring your knees to your chest and lift your hips to the level of your shoulders as you curl your body upward
2. Your back will be flat and horizontal with the floor; shoulders and hips will be on the same horizontal plane; knees will be over your chest and arms will be extended and straight
3. This position is known as the Tuck Front Lever
4. Reverse the motion as you inhale and return to the starting position
5. Repeat for a desired amount of repetitions per set

Body Parts Involved

1. Sides of your back (latissimus dorsi)
2. Back of your upper arms (triceps)
3. Stomach area (abdominals)
4. Hips (hip flexors)
5. Back of the shoulders (posterior deltoids)

Hanging Body Curls

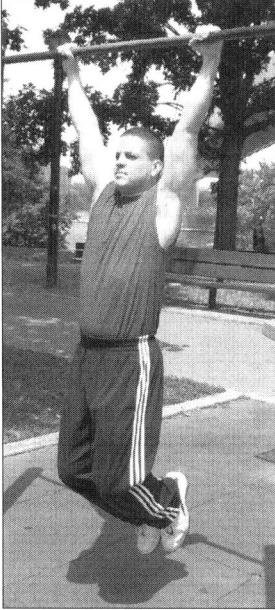

1

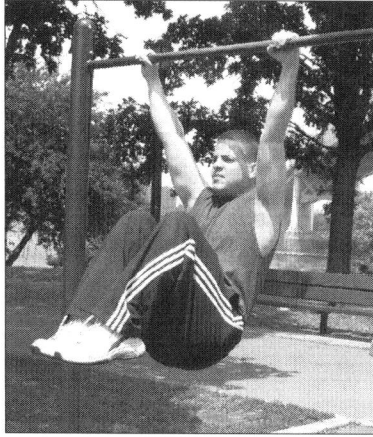

2

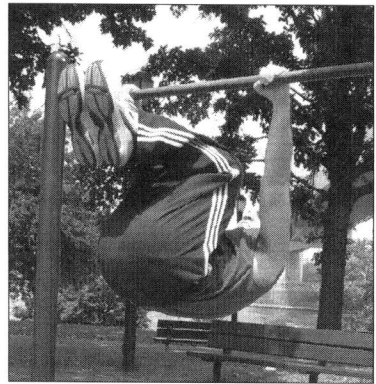

3

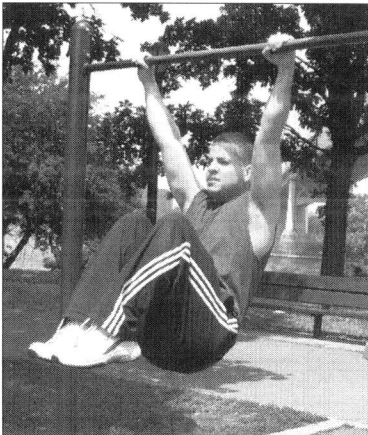

4

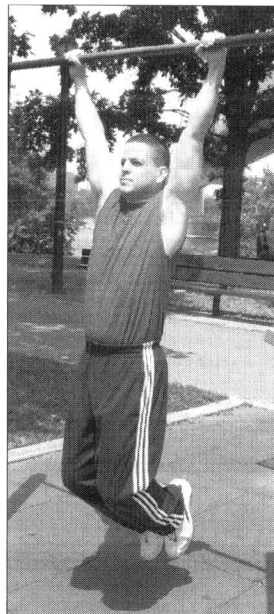

5

Hand Stand Body Curls

Starting Position

1. Assume a partial tuck planche position by:
2. dropping into a full squat and placing your hands on the ground, in front of your feet
3. resting your knees to the outside of your elbows
4. leaning forward until your feet are off the floor and your weight is on your hands
5. At this point, knees are resting on your elbows supporting some of your weight

Execution

1. As you exhale, continue to raise the hips until your upper body is in an up-side-down vertical position
2. Extend your hips and straighten your legs until you reach a full hand stand position
3. Both arms should be straight
4. Reverse the motion by first bending your knees as your lower them to the ground
5. Begin curling your body until your knees are resting on your elbows
6. Repeat for a desired amount of repetitions per set

Body Parts Involved

1. Shoulder (deltoids)
2. Upper back (upper trapezius)
3. Back of the upper arms (triceps)
4. Chest (pectorals)
5. Stomach area (abdominals)

Hand Stand Body Curls

1

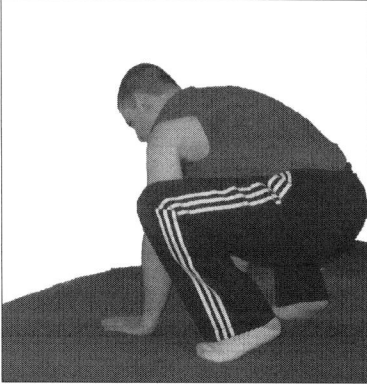

2

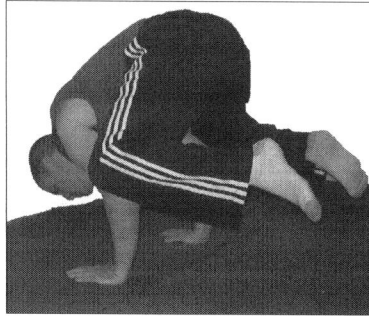

3

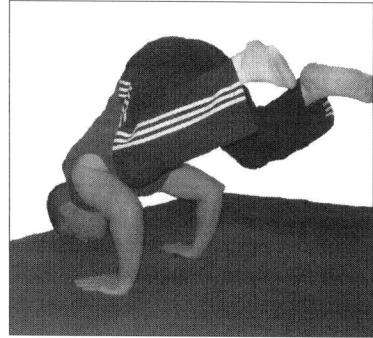

4

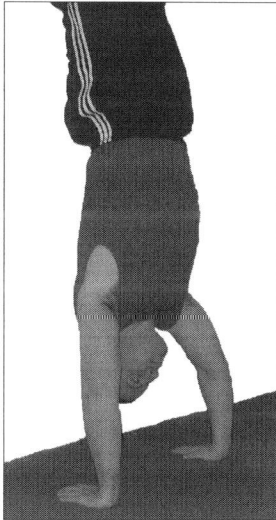

5

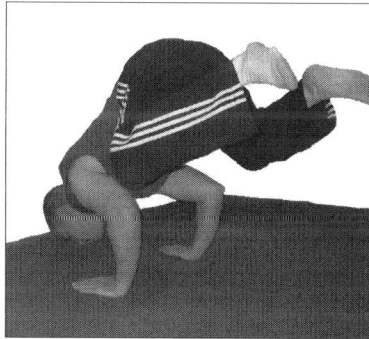

6

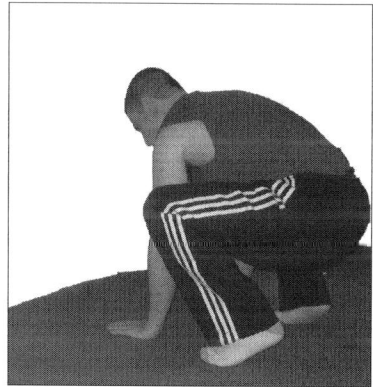

Sample *KineBody FSD* Routines

When performing any of the sample workout routines, or your own routines, keep the following chart in mind to determine what types of attributes your routine is training.

Weight	Attribute	Repetitions	# of Sets
Light	Endurance	12 - 20	1 - 3
Moderate	Hypertrophy	8 - 12	1 - 6
Heavy	Power/Strength	1 - 8	1 - 5

Remember, **KineBody's** bodyweight exercises can produce any of the above attributes as long as a state of muscular fatigue (or near fatigue) is reached during each set using the prescribed repetitions above. Rest periods in between sets can range from 30 seconds for endurance training, up to 2 minutes for hypertrophy training, to as high as 2 – 5 minutes for power training.

Any workout routine should be started with a light, 5 – 10 minute warmup that can include running in place, jogging, jump rope, shadow boxing, or anything that warms up the body and gets the heart pumping a bit.

In the following pages, you will see some quick examples of routines for novice, intermediate, and advanced fitness levels. Keep in mind to incorporate pushing and pulling exercises during your training. Don't get discouraged if you are just starting out. We all had to start from the beginning. This book was designed for all of us average people who want to get in shape, or are already in shape and want to try something different.

Novice Workout Routines

5 – 10 minute warmup

Routine #1

Standard 4 point Push Ups

Standard 2 - Arm **Chin** Ups

Abdominal Crunches

Supermans

Standard Squats

Jog in place for 2 minutes

(Repeat for 2 more sets)

Routine #2

Wide Grip 4 point Push Ups

Jog in place for 30 seconds

Standard 2 – Arm **Pull** Ups

Jog in place for 30 seconds

Wide Squats

Jog in place for 30 seconds

2 – Legged Calf Raises

Jog in place for 30 seconds

Oblique (Twisting Crunches)

Alternating Supermans

(Repeat for 2 more sets)

Intermediate Workout Routines

10 minute warmup

Routine #1

Side to Side, Top Starting, 4 point Push Ups

Horizontal Pull Ups (Knees over Chest)

Single Leg Forward Squats

Abdominal Crunches

Supermans

Lying Down Leg Lifts

Jog in place for 4 minutes

(Repeat for 2 more sets)

Routine #2

Hand Stand Push Ups

Side to Side, Bottom Starting Pull Ups

Jog in place for 2 minutes

1 Legged Squats (with chair sitting)

1 legged Calf Raises

Jog in place for 2 minutes

Pendulum Twists

Hanging Knee Lifts

Back Extensions

Jog in place for 2 minutes

(Repeat for 2 more sets)

Advanced Workout Routines

10 minute warmup

Routine #1

One Arm, 3 point Push Ups

Assisted, One Arm Chin Ups

Reverse, 4 point Push Ups

Horizontal Pull Ups (Knees over Hips)

Jog in place for 5 minutes

1 Legged Squats (Pistols)

2 Legged Curls (no arm assistance)

Reverse Leg Curls

Jog in place for 5 minutes

(Repeat for 1 more set)

Routine #2

2 Point Push Ups (No feet touching the floor)

Horizontal Pull Ups (Legs Straight)

Janda Sit Ups

Hanging Leg Lifts

Jog in place for 3 minutes

Hand Stand Body Curls

Hanging Body Curls

Back Extensions

Twisting Back Extensions

Jog in place for 3 minutes

Forward Leg Lunges

Chair Step Ups

Jog in place for 3 minutes

(Repeat for 1 more set)

Epilogue

I hope that you enjoyed this book and use the exercises presented as an everyday part of your training. No, one single book can ever contain all the fitness information needed to serve everybody, but my hope is that for the vast majority of everyday people who want to get healthy, feel good and look great, the **KineBody** series of books will provide a valuable alternative to other fitness programs.

So, keep training, take the exercises in this book, come up with your own routines, and make them your own.

Good luck with your training, make it a life long commitment, and take care.

For more information on **KineBody** books and other products, plus up-to-date workout routines, exercise examples, and information on the entire **KineBody** system, please visit:

www.KineBody.com

KineBody: your body ... your gym™

*E*d Aponte is the creator of the **KineBody** approach to fitness and wellness. A practitioner of the martial arts for over 20 years, Ed has traveled the world training with some of the best martial artists of their day. Ed has actively educated himself in various martial arts and health programs over the last two decades and has taught at Penn State University, placing second at the 1988 Isshinryu World Karate Championships, and earning the 1990 Outstanding Instructor Award. He has taught hundreds of clients in college settings, group settings, one-on-one training, and given various seminars to non-profit organizations, student groups, and households.

Ed holds a 2nd degree black belt through two Isshinryu Karate world organizations and has had varying degrees of supplemental training in arts such as Muay Thai, Kali, Arnis, Jiu-jitsu, Sambo, Russian martial art, and Jeet Kune Do. More recently, he completed a Personal Trainer curriculum through Equinox Fitness Clubs.

Ed has also written over one dozen articles for martial arts and fitness publications including **Black Belt** magazine, **World of Martial Arts** magazine, and **Dvizheniye: The Journal of Russian Martial Art**.

Through his years of active participation in the fitness and wellness industry, Ed still labels himself "just an average guy" and, thus, set about to create the **KineBody** system of **functional body development**. A system for the average person, for anyone and everyone to take and make it their own, **KineBody** consists of four training categories as follows:

- **Functional Strength Development**: the use of bodyweight exercises, leverage, and maximum tension to develop strength, conditioning, and endurance

- **Functional Flexibility & Joint Mobility**: muscular stretching and joint mobility drills to develop injury free movement throughout a greater range of motion

- **Functional Balance & Coordination**: incorporating static postures, footwork, and animated body mechanics to enhance balance and body awareness

- **Functional Sport Specificity**: putting it all together to enhance sport specific skills

Ed Aponte currently resides with his wife in New York City, working to develop the **KineBody** system of **functional body development**.

Made in the USA